PAIN
MANAGEMENT
AND YOU

*A Practical Approach to Living
with Chronic Pain and Illness*

PAIN
MANAGEMENT
AND YOU

*A Practical Approach to Living
with Chronic Pain and Illness*

Pain Management And You
All Rights Reserved © 2001, 2017 by Michael Gusack

No part of this book may be reproduced or transmitted in any form or by any means, graphic, electronic, or mechanical, including photocopying, recording, taping, or by any information storage retrieval system, without the permission in writing from the publisher.

ISBN: 978-1979276542

Printed in the United States of America

Contents

Preface ix
Acknowledgments xi
Introduction xiii
Part One: The Adjustment 1
The Slower You Go The Faster You Get There. 3
    Limitations 3
    Denial and Overexertion 4
    Frustration and Guilt 5
    Activity Broadly Defined 6
    Summary 9
And That's The Way It Is. 10
    Avoidance and Common Sense 10
    Acceptance 11
    Cultivating Readiness 12
    Gratitude and Creativity 14
    Ritual and Transformation 15
    Summary 17
Deservin's Got Uthin' To Do With It 18
    Faith 18
    Prayer and Gratitude 19
    Justice, Grace and Mercy 22
    Meditation 24
    Summary 25
Not Too Fast And Not Too Slow. 26
    The Measure of Worth 26
    Energy Conservation 28
    Not Too Slow 31
    Not Too Fast—Moderation 32
    Summary 35
It's Up To Who? 36
    Ignorance and Fear 36
    Knowledge and Understanding 38
    Information Gathering 40

  Mind and Body. 42
  Healthy Defiance 44
  Summary 46
Part Two: The Management **47**
What's So Funny? **49**
  Overdoing It. 49
  Laughter and the Body 50
  Humor and Detachment. 51
  Summary 54
If You "Feel" Like Doing It...Doing It! **55**
  Depression as Illness 55
  Challenging Our Depression. 57
  Roadblocks 59
  An Initial Plan 60
  Summary 62
It Just Isn't Worth It **63**
  Justified Anger 63
  The Consequences of Ignoring Anger 64
  It Just Isn't Worth It 66
  Listening to Anger 67
  Caution! Roadblocks Ahead! 69
  Summary 71
The Less Control We Need The More Control We'll Have **72**
  Fear and Uncertainty. 72
  Isolation 73
  Letting Go Daily. 75
  Worry. 76
  Worry Limiting Strategies 77
  Summary 80
Part Three: The Plan **81**
Turn Down The Volume **83**
  The Central Attitude. 83
  Stress Defined and Described 84
  The Relaxation Response. 85
  Approach and Intention 87

   A Few Specific Suggestions 88
   Summary 90
The Inevitable Is Coming! Better Plan For It. 91
   Balanced Optimism 91
   A Flare Is… 92
   Employment Considerations 92
   Family and Friends 93
   Relapse Is… 94
   The Nature of Change 95
   Warning Signs and the Plan 95
   The List 97
   Summary 99
Don't Just Survive…Thrive!. 100
   Stress Management 100
      Breath Awareness 101
      Autogenics 103
      Progressive Relaxation 104
      Insomnia 106
      Bubble Up 109
      The Word 109
      Pain 112
      Walking 120
      Conclusion 122
   Pain Management 122
      Chronic vs. Acute Pain 123
      TENS Unit 123
      Gentle Stimulation Alternatives 124
      Acupuncture 126
      Acupressure 126
      Stretching and Movement 127
      Biofeedback 128
      Miscellaneous 129
      Conclusion 129
   How We Change 130
      Opposition and Conflict 130

    Wait and See 131
    Awareness 132
    Staging the Process 132
    The Garden 133
    Summary 135
A Final Word. 136
About The Author 141
Resources. 143

PREFACE

OVER THE PAST nine years working both formally, and on a volunteer basis, I have served a diverse population of people coping with pain, stress, and chronic illness or injury. Personal experience with pain and several chronic illnesses, as well as clinical training have given me an intimate understanding of the challenges inherent in conditions that persist over extended periods of time.

Hypnosis training, along with years of involvement with meditation, yoga, Tai Chi, and Qigong have prepared me well for my work as a biofeedback therapist and counselor. These personal interests have enabled an integration of Eastern and Western healing traditions. I have blended these complementary traditions in a way that has empowered my clients to regain control of their lives as they develop skills and attitudes that best equip them to take advantage of life's opportunities for joy and satisfaction.

This integration is probably further enhanced by my academic background. I received my BA in Philosophy from Louisiana State University, and my MA in Counseling from the University of Colorado. I also did graduate work in Philosophy at Tulane University, and the University of Colorado. The impact of attitudes and beliefs on our daily routines has always been a strong interest, and thus a strength of mine.

As my clients have shared their struggles and triumphs with me, the seed that was planted after my hospitalization with Guillain-Barre' Syndrome has developed into this book. I am convinced that the message, and the approaches that have benefited my clients, will be useful to the millions of members of support groups and foundations established to cope with the problems associated with heart disease, diabetes, cancer, arthritis, and a multitude of other chronic illnesses. This book can also assist those of us over 45 who will easily relate to the challenge of some type of chronic problem… for a friend, if not for ourselves. The message here goes far beyond the confines of medical illness or injury per se', since it applies to pain that is spiritual, as well as physical in nature. Professionals too can again gain perspective, and find some useful and precise interventions that have been fired in the crucible of daily clinical practice.

My current practice and interests allow me to push the clinical envelope. I am working with biofeedback to facilitate and refine relaxation, meditation, and healing visualizations relative to physical and spiritual pain. I am exploring the potential benefits of brain-wave feedback. I am also incorporating treatment modalities such as photo-sonic stimulation, low frequency sound wave massage (based on research gleaned from studies of Chinese Qigong healing masters), and micro-current stimulation into my daily clinical practice. The task is, of course, to find what works for each of us. Attitude and belief have such a powerful impact on treatment outcomes…our mindset is often the key to the effectiveness of any given technique, any given device.

ACKNOWLEDGEMENTS

I WANT TO thank my wife Bert, and my girls Jamie and Natalie for tolerating the energy I've devoted to this project and to the odd hours that have often comprised my clinical practice and my training over the years. For all those…"When will you be home today?" and "When is your book going to be finished?"

Thanks to all those that read all or part of the manuscript…Allie Bailey, Bernard Pennington, Reg Altazan (the first), Donna Rigby, Michael DiMaria, Pat Brumfield, and my wife (who reviewed every revision!!) Their perspectives challenged me to infuse the text with as much clarity as possible and to structure it to be as useful to the intended audience as possible.

To Suzi Tucker the professional editor who followed the manuscript through two evolutions and provided invaluable suggestions regarding form, content and style despite the fact that her publishing house focuses primarily on professional trade books. And all this without charge! This was the labor of someone dedicated to her craft.

And finally to the countless individuals that have privileged me with the opportunity to accompany them for part of their healing journey as they taught me as much about their pain and illness as I was able to share with them.

INTRODUCTION

IF YOU HAVE ever had a problem with short attention span, then this book is for you. Historically, my memory has been unreliable at best. I remember some of the most bizarre trivia, and on the other hand, often have difficulty retaining what I would like to remember. As a coping strategy, I underline what I consider to be significant portions of articles or books that I read so that I can return to them, knowing that it would be an exception to the rule if I did remember them.

If you have been besieged by chronic illness or pain, you have probably found yourself forgetting where you placed the keys, or trying to remember what you were doing as you found yourself in a room at home without a clue as to why you were there. Stress takes its' toll. And longterm, chronic stress is the unavoidable consequence of long-term, pain and illness.

As you make adjustments to new situations and limitations, it's not surprising that you become distracted. When too much is heaped on your plate, something is bound to fall off. Concentration and memory are some of the first casualties. Accordingly, this book is organized in brief sections that provide opportunities for reflection that can carry you through your day. I have also included a brief summary at the end of each chapter to refresh your memory on its contents.

It is easy to lose trust and confidence in others and in ourselves as we experience, through our illness or our injury, a sense of isolation. It may seem as if our friends have deserted us. Our families may not seem to understand us. We may even feel that God has abandoned us, as if we are being punished for some misdeed of which we are unaware. Often our reaction is to isolate ourselves and cut ourselves off from contact with others. This further widens the gap, disconnects us, and leads us to become increasingly mistrustful and suspicious. It is probably true that we cannot "make" ourselves trust others when we have been let down, anymore than we can just "will" ourselves to renew a sense of self-confidence. But we can be open to that possibility and look for opportunities for the growth of trust and the rebuilding of self-confidence and assurance.

There are numerous well-written books and workbooks that address our need for understanding and direction in the healing journey toward recovery and acceptance. However, in my own personal recovery experience, as well as in my experience working with those who have chronic health problems, sometimes the anecdotes and research overwhelm us. Along the way to discovering the attitude and the perspective (if not the wisdom) that can meet our needs in the early stages of that journey, sometimes simplicity is preferable. This book can fill that gap, not only in terms of the format, but also in terms of a simple focus on attitude and expectations. I have found that the details often take care of themselves if we can just "get our minds right."

I have been in the counseling field for twenty-five years now, but perhaps the most significant part of my education relevant to this treatment is my personal experience with chronic illness and pain. I have had a kidney problem for the past seventeen years, which carries with it the potential for dialysis or transplant. I had a bout with GuillainBarre' Syndrome seven years ago (an auto-immune illness where the immune system gets confused and attacks the insulation around the nerves as if it doesn't belong there, leading to rapid numbing and paralysis). A car accident at age seventeen "sprained my spine", and my back has never been the same since.

There is always the danger of over-generalizing experience and assuming that the experience of others should be like one's own. However, I base what I am writing to you mainly on what has been confirmed for me through my work with others who have problems of a chronic nature. My clients do a good job of keeping me humble and honest. So let's get started!

Enjoy! Don't take it too seriously. And share this with some of your friends and family.

Part One

The Adjustment

THE SLOWER YOU GO THE FASTER YOU GET THERE

Limitations

MOST OF US have grown accustomed to an active life. When our abilities become limited, it often comes as quite a shock. There are those of us who are used to "hitting it at a hundred miles an hour" as we are in a state of perpetual motion, and optimum productivity. That old cliché, "The bigger they are, the harder they fall" holds true. The adjustment is most difficult for those of us who had grown accustomed to being energetic, successful, and the one on whom others depended. To our surprise, now it is we who need help. We are limited and encounter weakness for the first time in our lives.

We are in shock, disoriented and lost. It is like being dropped off on an entirely different planet where there are no familiar landmarks; the landscape is totally foreign to us. We were used to a fast pace. Our experience was, typically, that the harder we worked the more we accomplished and the more successful we were. We came to believe that we could do anything, we were invincible and invulnerable…virtually immortal. It never occurred to us that one day we could experience limitations on our daily activities. We became identified with the results of our work and play. We came to believe that our identity was completely defined by our accomplishments. There was no other. Being and doing were one and the same.

And thus, if we were not doing something…anything, we felt worthless, ashamed, and guilty.

When we were healthy many of us believed: "The faster you go, and the harder you work, the faster you get there." Well, now the rules have changed. Haven't they? We may not be able to do what we once could do; we may have to ask others for help; our life may be limited in countless ways. In fact, may be no area of our life that is not affected in some way. And this statement becomes increasingly accurate if the severity of our illness or injury becomes greater. We experience a confusing and often unnerving reality. "The slower you go, the faster you get there."

Denial and Overexertion

Well, exactly what am I trying to say? We need to learn that adamant refusal to accept the reality of our illness, our injury; our pain (whether it's physical, mental, emotional, or spiritual pain—and often it's all of these) just makes matters worse. When we become frustrated and push ourselves beyond our capacities, we pay for it. More pain, lower energy levels, loss of sleep, irritability, to name but a few are the price. Suddenly, our strategy, our style, for achieving satisfaction and realizing competence no longer works. Whenever we push ourselves beyond our limits, we discover that we don't awaken refreshed the following day. Before we know it, we're exhausted. As we struggle with these realities, we come to understand that "the slower you go, the faster you get there." We do not have to sacrifice the goal of achieving all of which we are capable, although clearly there may be things that we could once do that now we cannot. It is often possible to meet our goals, to complete the task in a way that does not exact a terrible price on our resources (e.g. sleep disruption or higher pain levels). We discover that if we can take it slow and easy, the job can, and will get done. We may have to do it incrementally; the job may take three hours instead of 15 minutes, it may have to be spaced across a period of several days, but the job can be completed. However true this may be, initially it will be difficult for us to find satisfaction and fulfillment in this slower pace. We are more likely to feel incompetent and frustrated.

Frustration and Guilt

Out of our frustration with this laborious process we may conclude that: "I just can't do anything anymore." We may isolate ourselves from friends and family due to embarrassment that we can no longer participate in activities as we once did. We struggle with guilt over the fact that we have to ask people for help. Family, friends, and coworkers are placed in positions where they are responsible for what we once could do effortlessly. Again we feel guilt. A friend recently asked me to consider this question. What exactly is it that we are guilty of? If we think about it, we can begin to realize that we really didn't do anything wrong. It's not as if we got injured or developed our illness on purpose. Most of my clients definitively proclaim that they wouldn't wish their situation on their worst enemy! Yes, our limitations clearly have an impact on those around us, but this wasn't planned, and was out of our control. We need to consider that if the onset of our condition was beyond our control (for obviously had we been in control, we would not be ill or injured), then it's not really our *fault*. We don't need to add to our problems by holding ourselves hostage with undeserved guilt.

When this shift in our perspective occurs when we are able to experience a sense of satisfaction, regardless of how our present achievements compare with our past accomplishments. Developing such an attitude diminishes our guilt. We can begin to reclaim our lives once we realize that we will never again operate at 100 percent of what our *old* Self was once physically capable. This doesn't require that we sacrifice Hope. In fact Hope is one of the essentials that fuels our capacity to persist in our pursuit of renewed happiness and vitality in our lives. It calls for our development of the ability to take life a day at a time without comparing it to the past. We are no longer wishing it wasn't so and looking back toward the pre-injury/illness days. We also learn to avoid worrying ourselves to distraction by wondering how much better or worse we'll be next week, month, or year. We admit that our crystal ball is too cloudy to provide us with a good view of what the future holds for us. The resulting present oriented outlook can open the gate to rebuilding our lives after our injury/illness.

All or nothing just doesn't work anymore. Because what that means is that we do a lot one day, and then we're in bed for the next three—or, if not in bed, certainly so exhausted and irritable that everyone is forced to suffer with us. Thus, the aftermath does not allow us the joy and satisfaction for which we had hoped, and we regret our behavior.

When we're finally able to acknowledge that there is something out of our control that's more powerful than we are, we begin to understand and appreciate the value of slowing down. And oddly enough, as we do slow down, tasks get completed. We are able to detach, to stand back and look at our experience in its entirety. It then becomes clear that in the space of a week, more gets accomplished if I do a little bit every day, versus spending half the week recovering from one days' Herculean effort. Satisfaction becomes possible when we realize that in order to do what we are now capable of doing, it will be useful to change our pace.

Activity Broadly Defined

However, we are only addressing physical activity at this point in our discussion.

These tasks to which I'm referring may be something, which is apparent to no one but us. For instance, chasing the elusive goal of acceptance and serenity is not a one-time event, but rather something that matures over time as the year's progress. Learning a new approach to our daily activities is a different kind of work, more subtle, but typically at least as intensive as any physical, objectively observable task we have ever done. This applies to every level of our being. Our injury/illness is with us every waking hour of the day…every sleeping hour as well, as our healing systems both physical and psycho-spiritual cope with the challenge. No one will ever witness this struggle, and we won't get paid for this work, but work it is nonetheless.[1] Interestingly, in the work lies the prospect of the relief we all seek from the unrelenting nature of our chronic problem.

The relief comes when we realize that we can continue to work toward being as active and productive as we can possibly be, but with a clear understanding of the context in which we move. The new context is that we're no longer 100 percent in the sense that there are certain physical limitations we now experience. We need to learn to function within these limitations. As we practice different behaviors with a fresh outlook this becomes our *new* Self. We can begin to experience joy and satisfaction as we did prior to our illness or injury. The accomplishments that now give us satisfaction may be radically different from our previous achievements, but they are no less meaningful or significant!

Perhaps there is a corollary to our "the slower you go" rule, namely that "less is more". Small accomplishments become large because of the time and effort we must now invest in them. It may take two days instead of two hours to mow the yard. Or it may take two hours rather than fifteen minutes to wash the dishes due to our limitations. Gratification is ours if we can claim our new Self.

---
1 The term "work" is meant to convey the fact that the changes we're pursuing require persistence and intensive effort.

Blindly fighting our pain, injury, or illness is fruitless. "The slower you go, the faster you get there" means that as we slow our pace, we will get results that are more immediate and long-lasting than our habitual pressured hard-hitting approach. We are coming to an understanding of the attitudes, expectations, and strategies that enable us to be as productive as we can be, and enable us to continue to explore our potential for growth. It's as if we are reborn via our injury/illness.

Summary

- The more accustomed we are to leading an active life, the more difficult it is likely to be to adjust to our present limitations.
- Refusal to accept the fact of our illness/injury leads to exhaustion and pain rather than to greater accomplishment.
- A realistic assessment of the limits of our control and responsibility can decrease feelings of guilt and worthlessness.
- Spiritual, mental, and emotional activity should not be construed as "doing nothing". Activity levels can be highly intensive in these realms.
- Coping with our illness/injury can be the hardest work we've ever done.
- The less we compare our present abilities to the past, the more content we will be. We will have a greater sense of accomplishment as well.
- A new Self can emerge when we acknowledge our limitations and set our pace and our goals accordingly.

This book is INTERACTIVE...

Ever have trouble just absorbing the impact of your pain and illness?

To get access to more resources visit...
http://michaelgusac.ibi3g.com/MYBK

AND THAT'S THE WAY IT IS

Avoidance and Common Sense

THERE ARE FEW things more annoying than someone telling us, or conveying the impression that we need to "Just stop whining and complaining, and learn to live with it." In our heart of hearts, we know that it is fairly good advice, but it also is advice that we're really not prepared to take. No one wants to believe that one's life has been irrevocably altered in ways so pervasive and powerful that one can only dimly express the impact of the illness or injury. None of us want to accept the harsh reality that this is not a temporary condition; that this is not going away. The natural reaction to extremely uncomfortable experiences is to run in the other direction. Certainly the natural reaction to being traumatized (and heaven knows chronic illness and injury is traumatic as its' reality impacts our lives) is to wish it wasn't so. In fact, it's likely to be our first reaction.

Avoidance may be the common sense approach, but the problem here with common sense and what is intuitive is that, for our particular situation, the rules don't apply. The natural order seems to have been disrupted. It has been pointed out to me by one of my colleagues (a Yale trained psychiatrist who hails from Eastern Europe), that the United States is one of the few countries on the planet that even has the concept "Pain Killer" as part of its' culture. Most other cultures acknowledge that joy and suffering are different sides of the same coin, that comfort and discomfort go hand in hand, that we have good days and bad days…"And That's the Way It Is." While suffering is certainly something we wish to transcend, it is understood as being "part of" vs. "opposed to" life. Death itself can be viewed as a part of life, rather than as the *end* of life. Thus a funeral could be a celebration of the memory of the departed, rather than a lamentation. Avoidance is one approach, but by no means the best.

Acceptance

What approach would be better? The answer is: "Acceptance." "Yuck!" you say? I appreciate your reluctance, because I'm aware that the word can conjure up images of settling for second best and giving up the fight. Let me describe what I have in mind. Perhaps a good way to define acceptance is by clarifying what it is not. Acceptance does *not* mean giving up hope. Acceptance does *not* mean that we have to decide that we "Just don't care anymore." To be apathetic is to deprive us of the strength and the energy we need to persevere during the formidable task of adjusting to a chronic situation. Since it *is* chronic (which by definition describes an injury/illness which has lasted for more than three months…briefer time frames are defined as "acute"), we need to be prepared for the duration.

Acceptance does *not* mean that "It's OK", or that we "Don't mind." Of course we mind. How could a long-term impairment possibly be "OK"? Not only would it be unrealistic to expect that we would adopt such an attitude, but it would not be useful to do so. "Well then, what would be useful? you may ask. We need to have a healthy dose of audacity and defiance to enable us to most effectively realize our current potential, so that we are not overly influenced by the opinions and expectations of others. If this is what acceptance is *not*, then what *is* it?

Acceptance is "giving in" without "giving up". This is often called "surrender". This amounts to acknowledging the limits of our control, and that our pain and illness is something, which has irrevocably altered our lives. Things will never be the same, and its not going away. If we can't get rid of it, it is possible to live *with* it. We can work in cooperation with the pain, the illness, as we listen to what it has to tell us. Perhaps, as ludicrous as this may sound, it's trying to *protect* us. While this may initially seem to contradict common sense, if we can indeed listen for the message, we may hear our body and mind telling us: "Take a break. Something is wrong. Take care of yourself. You don't have to feel guilty. We (body/mind) know you're doing your best. We need time to heal." None of us are *always* in control of our lives *all* of the time. The truth is that our pain and illness *will* take control at times. Perhaps it actually *should* take control. Our pain could provide a needed time out for repairs and protect us from further injury or exceeding our limits in a way that contributes to the progression of our illness.

Despite severe pain, or the flare-up of our symptoms, we don't *necessarily* have to be miserable. "Uncomfortable?" "Yes." "Miserable?" "No." While Hope is alive, we don't wait for a cure on some miraculous tomorrow. We take things a day at a time, an hour at a time, even a minute at a time, if necessary. And in so doing we are empowered. We discover the extent to which we *do* have control. As we listen and are guided by our body and mind, we discover what we *can* accomplish. And discovery is possible because we are paying attention and looking for learning opportunities.

Cultivating Readiness

What we are learning to do is to broaden our focus so that our vision is clear, and our perspective is complete. Given any particular circumstance relative to our illness/injury, will it be a *problem* or an *opportunity*? I've learned that, believe it or not, this perspective is a matter of choice. It's up to us to choose and it's as simple as accepting that responsibility and making the choice. Once the awareness and the readiness are there, then the choice is obvious and easy to make. The difficult part is, of course, cultivating the readiness and willingness to choose. Even when the choice is clear, we will not make it if we're not ready, if we're not prepared. Reading this book can be part of that preparation.

You may be thinking that reading this book alone will sufficiently prepare you…it's certainly a good beginning. To return to the concept of cultivating readiness, let us focus on the word "cultivating". Much like cultivating and tending a garden, readiness for change involves finding the balance between fertilizing, watering, and weeding the garden of healing acceptance.

Excess is as problematic as neglect. Too much water drowns the plants and allows disease to develop. Too much fertilizer will burn the plants. Similarly, we can try too hard, expect too much, and read to excess, thus confusing and frustrating ourselves. On the other hand, if we do not water sufficiently, the plants die. If we neglect to feed the plants, to fertilize them, they may not flower or bear fruit. This is analogous to a lack of effort, an avoidance of risk-taking and consequently neglecting to personally challenge ourselves to adjust to our injury/illness. We will remain stuck; we will not progress or be prepared to make the appropriate changes when the time is right.

Weeding out the old thoughts, attitudes and habits that interfere in our taking the most effective steps to further our health and healing is equally vital. Certainly the consequences of neglect are clear. Just as the weeds will choke out the garden and the plants will die, stubborn pride or unrelenting bitterness can easily interfere with any possibilities for constructive change and adjustment. It is also possible to exceed the limits of what will be helpful in this regard. Attempting too many changes and revisions at once will often lead to backsliding and regression. Gradual, incremental change is typically more permanent.

A balanced approach to readiness means we are open to growth and development without obsessing on the preparation. We're learning, reading, and challenging our beliefs and attitudes as we move toward our goal of making a healthy adjustment to our new circumstances. While we can be ready and we can be prepared, we can't *make* ourselves accept our injury/illness. This too is analogous to the plants in the garden. We can tend the garden, but we cannot dictate the day and hour on which the flower blooms. This is a matter of luck or, if you happen to take the spiritual view, an act of grace. We do the work of cultivating readiness, and acceptance will appear spontaneously.

Gratitude and Creativity

This does not discount or ignore our losses. We needn't pretend that everything is fine when it really isn't, but we are developing the ability to see the opportunities and possibilities contained in our circumstances and make use of them. We experience a sense of gratitude for what we still have, as opposed to grieving over what we have lost (although a true "Day At A Time", present orientation, also keeps alive the possibility that some of our losses can be recouped at some later date). While we have an awareness of our losses, we can nonetheless choose to experience an "Attitude of Gratitude". As we find ourselves able to feel grateful for what we have, we are experiencing one of the gifts that accompanies acceptance.

Acceptance also enables us to become more *creative* at finding solutions that allow us to do things that we had not previously considered possible. I'm reminded of a man in his 50's, with a back injury, who for over 5 years had hired someone to replace the cutting blades on his riding mower, because he couldn't crawl underneath it. One day it "occurred" to him that he could raise the tractor up with a winch high enough to expose the blades. He got himself a comfortable chair, and slowly, over a period of days, he was able to change the blades himself. The sense of release, freedom, and accomplishment he expressed was profound. We are not talking about a life free of conflict, but we are talking about a balance where joy and satisfaction are equally possible.

Ritual and Transformation

A group member, who had been a highly successful independent building contractor, once shared that each morning when he awakened and put on his work boots, he would tell himself: "I should be going to work today!" There are few among those of us whose work has been limited by our illness or injury that have not spoken those words…both silently and aloud. Here began the litany of guilt, shame, and worthlessness. Fortunately, however, his story does not end here. One morning, shortly after sunrise, which was when he normally awakened (just as he had all those years in the construction business), he took his boots outside in his back yard and burned them. This was his ritual of acceptance and surrender, and symbolized the fact that he would never again work as a construction contractor.

He described the relief he experienced when he burned those boots. He also said he experienced this act not only as liberating, but also as transforming. It had taken him years to reach this point in his adjustment to the limitations resulting from his injury. He had already gotten rid of his work tools by this point, but still persisted in telling himself that he should be going to work—with or without tools. Now he would awake to enjoy the sunrise. He had taken an important step in his journey toward spiritual and emotional healing and acceptance. In a very real sense, he had been reborn. Opportunities for growth and learning were again available.

There are difficult truths to confront when our lives are touched by pain and illness. However, life isn't over just because we may never be our old selves again. We can be transformed anew. Even though we are limited, we are not helpless. We need not be doomed to a life of existing to survive. Significant revision may be required, but happiness continues to be ours for the taking. In fact, our future may turn out to be brighter than it has ever been. Let's move on to explore the manner in which we can most effectively actualize that bright future.

Summary

- Avoidance may be the natural reaction to a chronic problem, but it is counterproductive. Unpleasant truths are best confronted.
- Acceptance does not require that we approve of our injury/illness. We can be defiant.
- Acceptance involves acknowledging the limits of our control, as we learn to live in the present.
- Chronic problems can be utilized for growth and learning. Problems can be transformed into opportunities.
- Cultivating readiness is like tending a garden. It requires a balanced approach.
- Focusing awareness on our assets enables creative solutions despite our limitations.
- A ritual of acceptance can open the door to a new happiness.

This book is INTERACTIVE...

Ever have trouble making peace with the facts?
To get access to more resources visit...
http://michaelgusac.odgi.net/MYBK2
There you can schedule a free 15-30 minute phone consult.

DESERVIN'S GOT UTHIN' TO DO WITH IT

Faith

PART OF WHAT can help us cope with chronic illness and pain is a certain faith regarding how things will turn out. If we are able to cultivate a belief and a conviction that, over time, in the larger perspective, things will work out, it will go a long way toward allowing us to begin to accept the reality of our limitations.

Many of us have had the experience that what initially seemed to be a problem, later (perhaps even years later) happened to have worked out for the best. We discovered that our perspective in the moment was not accurate when viewed over the course of time. What initially appeared unfortunate turned out to be, in fact, fortunate. Being able to see that larger perspective is a *great* asset in our journey toward acceptance and recovery. If we can believe that things happen for a reason, that there is a design, that the universe exists for a reason, then it's easier to learn how to transform problems into opportunities. We begin to look for the meaning of the challenge and what can be learned from it.

We can easily be overwhelmed by self-pity. There are certainly enough losses associated with chronic problems to exhaust anyone's lifetime allotment of misfortune. This often energizes an exaggerated sense of self-importance. However, it is difficult to feel sorry for ourselves if we have some sense that there is a purpose larger than ourselves in which we participate. While we do not necessarily have to believe in a world infused with purpose in order to experience acceptance and serenity, many of us will find it beneficial. I would say that it's worth trying on for size long enough to see if it fits—even if we have to "fake it" a bit in the beginning. "Well, that's a fine way to look at it," you may say. "But how are we to access this attitude?" "How are we really to feel that we participate in a fair and just world in the midst of our misfortune, our illness or pain?"

Let's examine a way of understanding the meaning of faith as a complement to the concept of belief. Faith can accommodate uncertainty. It does not require us to irrevocably and completely give our assent. We are allowed our doubts. If the word belief seems blind to the reality of your pain or misery, then attempt to trust and have faith in life's positive potentials despite *some* of the evidence to the contrary. Belief and faith can simply be different aspects of a spiritual sense of conviction. Doubt can be permitted for those with mature beliefs. Many are profoundly aware that it is possible to believe there is a larger purpose operating in our life and the lives of others. One way to access our personal beliefs, if we are religiously inclined, is through prayer.

Prayer and Gratitude

Prayer can be an activity that not only accesses our beliefs, but it can also establish a sense of connection that goes beyond our personal Ego. Prayer can take many forms—from calling out in a loud voice to God, to a prayerful attitude of receptivity, to whatever meaning

Spirit has to reveal to us. To pray for a cure is the natural reaction, but often a prayer for wisdom, understanding, and patience provides more relief as one seeks the optimal conditions for healing. If one is looking for meaning and understanding in daily experience, then the question becomes, "What can I learn from this?" as opposed to "How can I get rid of it?" What is it then that our illness/injury can teach us?

I often hear something to this effect: "I used to think that people who were sick or injured were weak, and now I'm one of them. Now I understand what it's like. I wouldn't dream of saying some of the things I once said." I have noticed that when we take strength (i.e. physical and spiritual) for granted, we come to believe that affliction with disease or injury can only happen to others, it can never happen to us. "They" are weak. *We* are strong. Very often others see us in this light as well. They saw us as strong and dependable; "the rock" on which they relied and from which they sought support. To learn that we too can be weak, often vulnerable and therefore human is a valuable lesson. This is a highly significant part of what our chronic problems can teach us.

We learn that there are circumstances out of our control; that we are not totally in control. We learn that there are limits to what willpower can accomplish and our determination can overcome. Determination, clearly, is an important part in the recovery of our ability to persist in learning the changes in attitude that facilitate healing, recovery, and joyful satisfaction. Learning that we do not have as much control as we would like to think can be a sobering discovery. At the same time, it can be a lesson that provides relief and freedom, freedom from the exaggerated selfimportance of self-pity, and the freedom to begin seeing a larger perspective, the "God's eye view".

When we begin to see this larger perspective, we begin to think about how we can contribute to the quality of life for others, and perhaps our community at large. I would suggest that this is actually another form of prayerful activity, which will access our experience of life's larger purpose. That is to say, an act, which offers service to another human being in need, can be a prayer. It affirms our kinship with a larger community, and the worth of our fellows. It is a prayer that honors our connection with Life itself, the universe, or God, as we understand him. We might, in fact, actually feel grateful and fortunate if we were, for example, doing some volunteer work at a nursing home or a surgical recovery unit at a hospital as opposed to sitting at home immersed in our grief and boredom.

The gratitude to which I have referred in this book is another aspect of our experience of our spirituality (that sense of connection with others, with our surroundings and circumstances, if not indeed with the universe itself). Certainly surrender of our sense of Ego, of separate individuality, (that experience of our separateness from Nature, God, and our fellow man) is an act that frees us to revision our Selves, to see ourselves anew. We are better able to appreciate the health we have and what our potential for the future can be, in spite of the limitations that force us to explore new strategies for accomplishing familiar tasks and find new interests that accommodate our current abilities. To develop gratitude, as well as faith, creates the perspective that things will, in fact, work out for the best. Then we need not worry so much (although worry is, of course, to some degree unavoidable). We can thus focus on that over which we in fact *do* have control (for example, our attitudes and how we respond to our reactions).

Beyond prayer, and how we use it to nourish a sense of faith and meaning in our lives, it is also important to nourish our spiritual selves by looking for opportunities to build trust and confidence in ourselves, and others. This is a variation on the theme of faith with perhaps a more personal frame of reference. Maybe trust is just another word for faith. This may be a partial explanation for why I am so often told by my clients that their participation in group counseling and education is the most helpful part of their treatment. Group activities with people with similar challenges lends us an opportunity to be helpful to others (the service to which we have been referring), and to trust that there are those who care, understand, and can be trusted.

Justice, Grace and Mercy

An understanding that can be useful in our relationship with the larger reality, and with God, has to do with our perspective regarding how one is rewarded for his or her efforts. This brings to mind a theme from a movie I saw during a recurrence of some of the symptoms of my GuillainBarre'. This was about a year or so after recovering from its most debilitating effects. The scene comes from a western entitled "The Unforgiven". In the scene the anti-hero is about to take the life of the corrupt sheriff who has just brutally killed the hero's close friend. As the sheriff is confronting his death, he remarks that he is just concluding building the house on which he has been working for some time, and that he "Doesn't deserve to die" when he's so close to completing his long sought after goal. The character responds that "Deservin's got nuthin' to do with it." He then finishes off the sheriff.

There are numerous themes of separation from self and others and the search for redemption during this movie. The comment about "deserving" struck a chord with me. I thought of the fact that the visitations of fortune and misfortune are unpredictable and often seem unwarranted. Regardless of how virtuous we are, or how diligent or conscientious we are, this is no guarantee against illness, injury, or disaster. I had been doing a good job of behaving myself by following my neurologist's recommendations for maintaining my health. Nonetheless, despite my diligence, I had to watch my health deteriorate as the numbness and tingling began to return.

This reality doesn't feel "fair" *because it isn't fair*, at least if we are referring to getting our "just reward" for our efforts. Now, this doesn't have to leave us with a sense of hopeless despair in a meaningless universe. It is simply an acknowledgement of a reality that then releases us to focus, not on whether justice is being done, but to courageously confront the mysteries of our often uncertain and unpredictable existence. We can then take responsibility for doing our best to get back on track and create the optimal conditions for our healing and recovery. We continue to follow the physician's advice and do whatever else contributes to reclaiming our previous level of functioning.

In the Christian framework, it is understood that Salvation has nothing to do with "deserving", in the sense that there is something one can do to deserve it. Salvation is a gift. So in the midst of our illness, injury, and pain, we can gain a sense of being gifted with mercy and grace even in the face of misfortune, if not tragedy. If we neither "deserve" some of what we have been *given*, nor "deserve" to have some things taken *away*, and then we can let go of ruminating over whether life is fair, and focus on the moment's opportunities. This is well encapsulated in this brief quote from a sermon I once heard in church:

> Yesterday is History
> Tomorrow is a Mystery
> Today is a Gift
> That's Why They Call It
> "The Present"

We can focus on the wonder and opportunities of the day, in spite of life's unfairness and our losses and limitations. We can appreciate what we have and thank God for the gifts with which we *are* blessed such as our family, our intelligence, our compassion, and the list goes on. And perhaps we eventually discover that these lessons we are learning enrich our lives in ways we cannot imagine and which clearly we would never have encountered were it not for our illness or injury. We begin to again feel connected to our world.

Meditation

Meditation is another strategy for developing this sense of connection. It too is a kind of prayerful, receptive attitude. In meditation, we may simply adopt a quiet, watchful, and attentive attitude as the mind chatter, the internal dialogue fades, and then is extinguished. We may use a particular technique, such as focusing our attention on a candle flame, our breathing, or a repetitive phrase. This helps quiet our mind and open our awareness. It is a state where we are mindful of the full presence of the immediate moment. The term "mindfulness" is often used in this context. Meditation helps create a frame of reference where selfimportance is unfitting. The sense of Self dissolves. We experience a sense of connectedness with our surroundings and our social environment. And there are other ways of cultivating this meditative experience of connection and transcendence.

For some of us, nature, and our presence in nature can be our meditative connection. Another simple way to access this sense of connection with nature is through walking. While walking we can be in natural environments that are relaxing and energizing. They remind us that there is more to the world than ourselves. In spite of our pain or illness we have a willingness to give, to share our time and our Selves with others. Sharing is another entrance to that feeling of connection with something greater than ourselves. When we let go of our self-absorbed, narcissistic outlook, are we able to experience a sense of community, a sense of something greater than ourselves of which we can be a part and from which we can draw strength.

Summary

- Faith that things will work out in the long run is a great asset in our adjustment to pain and illness.
- Prayer is a multi-faceted activity that can put faith into action. Service oriented activities can be prayerful as well.
- Gratitude is experienced as our perspective expands beyond our personal circumstances.
- Healthy behavior does not guarantee health, but must be pursued nonetheless.
- We cannot fully protect ourselves from misfortune, but we are fortunate in that we are graced with various blessings as well.
- The present moment is the aspect of time that is most fully real. In comparison with the past and the future the present is a gift.
- Meditation can help us develop a sense of connection with life and transcendence beyond our suffering.

This book is INTERACTIVE...

Chronic pain and illness can challenge our faith in GOD, in others, in Life itself. To get access to resources that lead to the sense of control that can restore your faith visit...

http://michaelgusac.ibi3g.com/MYBK3

NOT TOO FAST AND NOT TOO SLOW

The Measure of Worth

HOW CAN WE find a balance in our activity level? The concept of pacing addresses this question. How much is too much, and how much is not enough? As our illness or injury initially affects us, we often find ourselves making comparisons between the present and the past. Our abilities prior to our injury are the standard against which we measure what should, or should not, be our current ability level. We are challenged every day, perhaps even every hour, with decisions regarding which tasks we should attempt.

When we experience new limitations on our activity levels, we need to learn to pace ourselves within these limitations. The initial challenge will be making the decision to take a break, and being aware that a break, in fact, is needed. Our tendency will be to exceed our limits (pretending that things are no different than they ever were) and attempt to carry out any given activity as we normally would. However, in so doing we will limit our recuperative abilities, decrease our energy level, and probably increase our pain level. When we are accustomed to easily completing a task at one sitting, we find that it is exceedingly difficult to slow down and gain a sense of satisfaction from the completed task. If it takes us three hours to complete what previously took 30 minutes, it just doesn't feel like the same piece of work. It doesn't feel worthwhile. And not only does the task seem less worthwhile, we often feel less worthwhile as a person. We feel incompetent despite the final outcome.

The fact that someone who was not by our side the entire time, seeing the completed task, would simply credit us with a job well done, does not console us. *We* are aware that something is different, and *that* is what most impresses us.

Let me suggest a way of thinking about our activity level that can increase our sense of satisfaction, and enable us to take the time we need to comfortably complete any given task. There was a time when I could trim the ten-foot hedge that runs along the side of my property in about three hours. However, since having developed Guillain-Barre', it has taken as long as three days to do the same task, given limited levels of strength and stamina. Yet, I would like us to consider this: If it takes three days to complete a task that once took three hours, not only is the task *as* worthwhile as it ever was, it is even *more* worthwhile now.

What course of reasoning is this? Consider that if the job costs more effort and time, then perhaps it's worth more. If it now takes you three hours to wash the dishes, whereas it previously took you three hours to clean the entire house, then both of these tasks, given your energy output, are equally worthwhile. Obviously, we don't have as much to show for it, but it certainly cost us just as much in terms of what we invested in the project. Our assessment of the worth of our effort often relates to the value we place on how other people evaluate our accomplishments. If we are not exclusively focused on what others think, then we can take personal responsibility for meeting our need to feel worthwhile. We needn't expect others to infuse us with this feeling of worthiness. As a result we can take satisfaction in our day-to-day activities. You may initially find yourself under the impression that you are simply lying to yourself about the worth of your work. This would be a natural reaction, but challenge yourself, experiment, and see if this approach doesn't begin to ring true.

This reminds me of a comment I once heard. We are "Human beings", not "Human doings". The meaning intended is that what defines us as individuals, is not solely limited to what we produce. Our worth goes far beyond this. We need to consider that *regardless* of what we *do*; we are, in every other respect, the same person. For instance, if you were responsible and industrious before your injury or illness, you are still that person with those very same qualities. Despite being unable to produce some of the results that would demonstrate these personality traits, they continue to be there.

You may feel worthless, but that feeling is attached to the 'human doing' perspective. Most of us learned to measure our worth by the size of our paycheck and our accomplishments. We learned that we are what we *do*. Many of us also learned to focus on the opinions of others as the primary source of our worth. If we approved of an activity, and someone else did not approve, then often his or her opinion carried more weight than our own assessment of the value of that activity. But we are actually the best judges of the value of our achievements, since beyond the obvious outcome only we can know how much effort any given activity requires. It is my belief, however, that we are more than simply what we physically do. We need to cultivate faith in our judgment. We must set new standards as we evaluate our worth and the worth of our activities.

Energy Conservation

Another perspective or attitude relevant to pacing is energy conservation. An illustration that can be helpful in conceptualizing this attitude is one that I came across during my education as a trainer for the Lupus Foundation of America. Imagine that your energy is like a bowl full of marbles. Your day begins with a full bowl. Each activity during the day will cost you some marbles. Some activities cost more than others do. Waking up may cost you two marbles, while fighting it out with the boss might cost you ten. The goal of energy conservation is that by the end of the day, you still have a few marbles left in reserve…even when your head hits the pillow at the end of the day.

This was not necessary when you were healthy. But once affected by illness and injury, even at night while asleep, your body and your unconscious mind are still coping with that reality. As a result, even if you do a good job of managing your energy, so that you run out of marbles just as your day concludes, the bowl will not be full when you awaken the next morning. Energy was being expended throughout the night. And before you know it, as the days, weeks and months progress, you wake up one morning, and there's nothing left in your bowl, you're "running on empty".

And in reference to running…consider the marathon runner; if the runner doesn't pace, the race is not run. Exhaustion ends the race prematurely. You actually need to have some energy in reserve for completing the race, for getting you through the night. The goal is to conserve our energy by the minute, the hour and the day. We do not want to find ourselves midway through the day, having "lost our marbles" (i.e., our *energy* marbles).

In common parlance, losing one's marbles connotes losing control of one's emotional and mental faculties. This becomes a far greater risk when our energy level is at low ebb over an extended period of weeks and months. I would suggest that "losing it" emotionally or mentally is often primarily a matter of being so exhausted at every level of our being that our normal coping abilities are no longer sufficient. We have exceeded our limit. This is quite frightening, and quite surprising for one who is accustomed to coping effectively, but in more ways than not, it could also be considered a natural reaction to being chronically exhausted and overwhelmed.

Although it is true that many activities require energy and drain us, there are also activities that put energy (marbles) back into our bowl. A visit with a friend, a walk on the beach, and reading a good book are some examples. Meditating is another example. Even if no one sees the activity in which we are engaged, please remember that it is activity nonetheless. This is an important consideration as we gauge the worth of our day, and the extent to which our satisfaction is justified.

Physical activity, let us be reminded, is simply one aspect of activity. Energy is expended in many other ways as well: spiritual activity, emotional activity, and mental activity to be specific. We have all experienced, at one time or another, feeling exhausted after thinking through a problem or getting upset. That can be the evidence to which we refer as we begin to understand that there is much more to the world than meets the eye when examining energy output. When we berate ourselves because we're "doing nothing", we would benefit from understanding that we are active throughout the day regardless of how it appears to the observer. In fact, I would challenge you with my understanding, or belief, that you are in fact working harder now than you ever have in your life. This applies whether your illness or injury is so debilitating you cannot work (for a day, or permanently), or whether it requires that you make adjustments to your style of living on a day-to-day basis. We are constantly challenged to maintain a level of awareness that allows us to make useful adjustments to the dictates of our illness and injury as we go through the day. Managing our energy, disease, pain, or injury is a twenty-four-hour-a-day task. We never had a friend who was so close, who kept us in such good company as our pain or illness. And I don't mean to be ludicrous by using the words "Good Company". It *is* possible to view our challenges as friends. But that's another discussion.

Not Too Slow

Pacing is learning not only how to take breaks, but also how to maintain an adequate level of activity in whatever realm of which we are speaking (i.e., physical, emotional, mental or spiritual). Learning to take breaks will be the first lesson of pacing for most of us. However, as we progress, we also come to understand that too little activity can be equally destructive, if not devastating. Pacing is not a way to figure out how to make excuses for being unproductive. It is not a strategy for justifying laziness. Again, the point of pacing ourselves is to develop a strategy for being as active and productive as we can possibly be. Surprised? For most of us, when we think about the word pacing, it has to do with taking a break, but it also has do with reclaiming control in our lives which requires energy and persistence.

It is important that we maintain our current repertoire of activities to the best of our ability in order to maintain our range of motion, strength, and stamina. There may be certain activities that we are no longer able to carry out. However, activities in which we *are* currently able to comfortably participate will become uncomfortable, if neglected. Remember that this applies to activities of any kind, regardless of our health status. For instance, if I haven't thrown softball in the past year, and I then spend an afternoon throwing the ball for hours, I wouldn't be surprised if my arm ached the following day. We are all likely to experience that a long period of inactivity will trigger increased pain levels. When injured or ill the length of time will, of course, vary. For some of us, 20 minutes of inactivity will require a postural change. Or we may have to constantly shift from standing, to sitting to lying down in order to manage our pain.

If you favor your pain, those muscles will become de-conditioned, out of shape. Virtually everyone's first reaction is to ease up, to require less from the area of our body that hurts. Unfortunately, over time, the muscles can lose mass and elasticity. Then they have to be retrained to once again carry their normal workload. Hence the phrase "use it or lose it".

Pain levels increase, not only relative to how our body responds to inactivity, but also in response to how preoccupied we tend to become with our pain to the exclusion of all else. The more you watch your illness and your pain, the larger it tends to become. And this is *real*.

Numerous research studies have demonstrated that physiologically, in terms of muscle tension levels, release of neuro-chemicals, and other phenomena, that we become sensitized to our pain. It is important that we begin to challenge ourselves to be active, in order to maintain our strength, and our stamina.

On a different note relative to retaining our current abilities and skills, let's briefly consider the examples of prayer and relaxation practice. If we do not maintain an active regimen of prayer or relaxation, we can lose touch with these skills, these abilities. And then, simply because we've not been doing it for a while, we may experience emotional or spiritual discomfort when we revisit these activities. It's not necessarily going to be physically uncomfortable, but discomfort it is nonetheless. It will feel foreign and require time and effort to regain the skill we once possessed. This is not like riding a bike. Practice is required to maintain our facility with these types of activities. Staying active on these various activity levels is perhaps less of a challenge than stopping to take breaks, but nonetheless is important to bear in mind.

Not Too Fast—Moderation

Maintaining our activity levels becomes more challenging however when as a result of overdoing it, we experience higher pain levels. Then, with regret and disgust, we may go overboard in the other direction, and simply avoid that type of activity altogether. "I'll never rake that yard again!" we proclaim. This is a big mistake. When we overdo it we may have to wait three days to return to normal activity levels, but we can learn from this experience. It becomes exceedingly obvious that there must be a better way, a less painful way to approach maintaining our activity level. What we will discover through repeated incidents of overextending ourselves, is that we will actually get more accomplished if we engage in activities in increments, one segment at a time. By taking breaks, pacing ourselves and thus maintaining a balance of activity as we go through the day, we actually get more accomplished. As we see the results, we experience increased levels of satisfaction. We feel more worthwhile.

The Greek philosopher Aristotle affirmed the general principle: use moderation in all things. Moderation is a theme throughout this book. The challenge for us with pacing, as with almost every other adjustment to our new reality, is to find the balance. We need something in the middle, not to the extreme in either direction—not too much, and not too little. One thing that can help you do this is the knowledge of *how* to go about pacing yourself.

An excellent strategy is suggested in a workbook by Margaret A. Caudill, M.D., Ph.D., entitled, *Managing Your Pain Before It Manages You*. The strategy involves a self-assessment in which we first identify our typical pain level. This is the "baseline".

Then we identify how long we can engage in a particular activity before it significantly increases our pain level. We then identify how much break time is required to return to our baseline level of comfort. For example, if you wash the dishes for ten minutes, and your pain level goes from a 5 to a 7, then how long does it take before it goes back to 5 (baseline)? If it takes 20 minutes to return to baseline, then that is your break time.

We could also use this strategy to assess and manage our energy level. Lupus patients, for instance, are often confronted with the problem of conserving energy, as are chronic fatigue patients. Depression could also challenge us to conserve what little energy we may have. We would then explore how much energy we expend in a particular activity. And when our energy drops two levels, then its time for a break. Now with energy, a break may or may not replenish some of those "lost marbles", but it can at least help us guard against energy depletion.

While there may be some variation depending on whether we are having a good day or a bad day, in general, we can get a sense of how long we can be engaged in a particular activity before a break is required. And that break need not be just twiddling our thumbs, wasting time. We can engage in activities such as meditation, calling a friend on the phone, reading our Bible, and listening to music and so on. These break-time activities can actually re-energize us, as well as decrease our pain levels. It *is* possible to put marbles back in the bowl. It need not lead to doing "nothing", if such a thing even exists.

Our initial reaction to chronic illness/injury is to avoid the accompanying discomfort, to try to ignore our pain and our limitations. To journal and track our pain and discomfort may be counter intuitive, but the results speak for themselves. How can we effectively manage something about which we are ignorant? We must educate ourselves and become literate in the language of our injury/illness, in the daily context in which we must function. This is not hyper-vigilance or morbid preoccupation. This is intelligent preparation. If we listen to our illness/ injury, we may discover it will be more responsive and manageable as a result. So explore this thing called *pacing*. Give it an honest effort. Find the balance for *your* activity level. And read on.

Summary

- The degree of effort a task requires is a measure of its worth.
- We are human "beings", not human "doings". We are more than what we physically achieve.
- Take care that you don't "lose your marbles" (energy marbles). Energy conservation is vital.
- We are working harder now than we ever have worked in our entire lives...we're just not getting paid for it.
- It is important that we remain as active as possible. Inactivity can be just as problematic as overdoing it.
- The choice to take breaks will lead to greater overall levels of productive activity.
- Lack of awareness of the connections between pain, energy level and our daily activities will ultimately result in more pain and greater limitations.
- Seek balance and moderation in your daily routine.

This book is INTERACTIVE...

Ever have trouble slowing down and pacing yourself? To get access to more resources to help with this visit...
http://michaelgusac.odgi.net/MYBK4

IT'S UP TO WHO?

Ignorance and Fear

AT BEST, THERE'S a world of uncertainty associated with chronic health problems. The future holds many unanswered questions. The importance of understanding all that we can about the nature of our illness or injury cannot be overstated. We need to look to the health care provider as our teacher and our ally in this regard. I encourage you to ask the physician, the massage therapist, the acupuncturist, the biofeedback therapist, the physical therapist, the nurse, or other health care professionals for the details regarding your situation.

Ask for their understanding of the basic characteristics of your problem, and the anticipated benefits, and/or effects that will be obtained from any particular procedure, be it diagnostic or treatment oriented. Ask them to suggest books or other publications you might read to enhance your understanding. You might also ask them to recommend any Internet web sites that they believe could be informative or supportive. If you're not currently computer literate, it's easier than you think to utilize this tool for research. It just takes some time and effort. If you don't own a computer, ask a friend who does for a little help…or try your local library or college. Such steps help you gain a sense of mastery over your circumstances as you begin to grasp the nuances and subtleties of your illness or injury.

Now while there's a part of us that is driven to pursue this educational quest, there are other forces at play as well. In the early, acute, stages of our illness/injury we're waiting for our problem to go away (as it always had in the past). We are accustomed to coping with the 3-day flu, a cold, or a broken bone. In these circumstances we could usually predict the length of time required to return us to a healthy level of functioning. And for those of us who rarely, if ever, had to consult with a physician for *any* medical concern, we will probably find ourselves thinking, "I can't believe this is really happening." We're virtually in a state of shock. We're waiting to awaken from the dream, if not indeed the nightmare. But, as the condition progresses beyond the first three months (the clinical definition of "chronic") regardless of our past history, the reality of our situation begins to sink in. We may become anxious or fearful, as we ask ourselves certain questions. What might we find out when we do get the details? What if we're told that we're going to have to "learn to live with it", that it's not going to get any better, or that it will likely get worse? We might have to confront the fact that our life has been irrevocably changed.

When I first learned of my kidney disease, I did a fair amount of information gathering. I asked my nephrologist a lot of questions and thought I was being quite thorough. My wife, coincidentally, happened to be Head Nurse for the Kidney Transplant Unit at the University of Colorado Medical Center when I received my diagnosis. She was extremely helpful and informative. I certainly had plenty of information at my disposal. But it was not until almost a year later that I straightforwardly asked my physician about my prognosis. It took a lot of "getting used to" before I was ready to risk not only hearing that it was never going to completely go away, but also to risk hearing what the long term impact might be. Might I need to prepare for the likelihood of dialysis or kidney transplant?

Be aware that fear, denial, shock, grief, anger, and resentment, can all interfere with our willingness and ability to learn. While lack of knowledge, understanding, and information may cast us adrift, at the same time, privately we hope that "No news is good news". If we don't hear anything bad, then at least there's the possibility of complete and total recovery. Nobody's going to tell us that our time is limited. I believe Shakespeare wrote "*If* ignorance is bliss, then 'tis wise to be ignorant". That's a big IF! Given our circumstances, ignorance carries anything but bliss as its consequence…at least in the long view.

Knowledge and Understanding

Now the pace of medicine is often so fast that the providers are simply trying to get to the next person on their schedule as quickly as they can. As a consequence, the time it takes to establish a dialogue is often elusive. Many of us have had the experience of waiting lengthy periods in the waiting room (aptly named), only to be rushed in and out of the exam room with no time to ask that question we had prepared for the doctor. In fact, sometimes it all happens so quickly, we can't even remember what we wanted to ask in the first place. Some if not many of us have also had the experience of forgetting the provider's recommendations the instant the clinic's doors closed behind us.

In contrast, there are those times when we have to wait weeks and months to get the results of a diagnostic procedure we've undergone. There may have been times when we've waited a seeming eternity to experience the potential benefits of a new treatment approach. However, regardless of whether things are moving too fast or too slow, pursuing the information is the task. The point is, if we do not actively seek information and understanding, it may be a long wait before it comes to us, if it ever does.

It is not unusual in the course of my work with clients to encounter people who cannot describe the details of their illness or injury, or the accompanying treatment. This surprises me at times. But then I consider that we prefer to trust the professionals to do their jobs and give us the results for which we hope. This is much the same attitude we invoke when we take our car to the repair shop. We don't necessarily need to be a mechanic or know the workings of a machine to reap the benefits of the service, do we? And do we really need to be a neurosurgeon or an orthopedist? Do we really need to know all the details to which they must attend to get better ourselves? Of course not! However, in this instance we need to learn as much as possible. If our body/mind, our machine, is not functioning properly on a chronic basis, there are limits to what the experts can do. Perhaps this is because the mechanism of this machine involves the complexities of spirit, emotion, and mind as well as the functioning of the body. Chronic illness, injury, and pain go far beyond nerve, muscles, bones, and fluids. It's also a matter of perceptions, expectations, and attitudes.

Now once again, we may be ambivalent in our wish to learn of the diagnosis. We may then feel obligated to certain actions and encounter certain responsibilities in our recovery (limitations, restrictions, and attitude revisions may be required). Whether we like the news or not, and whether we choose to act on that knowledge, it is nonetheless important to understand how we can best participate in our own recovery. It is important for us to understand precisely both what is required, and what should be avoided relative to furthering our rehabilitation. As we are equipped with greater understanding, we can better develop realistic expectations for our daily routine and plans.

In some ways knowledge is power. The more we understand, the more tools we have in our recovery kit. The more actively we participate in our recovery, the more effective and successful it is likely to be. There's a saying that goes "It works if you work it". This is true for the healing journey of those of us challenged by chronic injury and illness. This is how we create the optimal conditions for becoming as active and productive as we can.

Information Gathering

What then is a good strategy for acquiring this information? I highly recommend going to any appointment you have regarding your condition with pencil and paper in hand. *Prior* to your appointment, write down a list of any questions or concerns you have about your treatment, diagnosis or prognosis and be sure to take them along with you. Then prioritize that list so that if there's not enough time to answer all your questions, you'll get the vital issues covered. You may want to have a copy that you can give to the health care provider with whom you're meeting so that both of you can review them together during your appointment.

My cousin exemplifies the wisdom of this approach. She told me that she had been to numerous doctors before finally being diagnosed with Crohn's disease. She said that the physician who did diagnose her was the first to have the benefit of her handwritten list of each and every symptom she had experienced. After reading the list, he announced his suspicion regarding her disease, and the diagnosis was confirmed with tests the very next day. Her search had finally ended.

You can also benefit by taking notes *during* your meeting. Much of this information is emotionally charged. Anxiety can easily erase your memory. If you take notes, you can refer to them later without needing to wrack your brain in an effort to remember detailed recommendations. This will also enable you to intelligently relay the details of your visit to friends and family. You may even want to invite them to an occasional appointment for support, perspective, and twice the memory.

To bring a notepad into the office suggests that we have a right to take notes, to take the provider's time. I certainly declare that right. We are entitled. Just remember that healthcare providers are, in fact, "providers". A service is being offered. As much as we may develop trusting relationships with those with whom we associate in our care and treatment, they typically are not our "friends", and they are certainly not simply doing us a "favor", rather they are paid to provide a service. If we are not satisfied with the service, we have the right to express our dissatisfaction. If we disagree, we have the right to speak up. If we want another opinion, we are entitled to at least ask. Such expressions and requests need not be interpreted as an insult; it's simply a matter of making well-informed decisions that may well impact the rest of our lives. There certainly are other areas of our lives where we get more than one estimate before we get the job done (e.g. roof or car repair). If we don't like the work, we probably won't continue to use their services.

I am not suggesting an adversarial posture. More often than not we will be immensely appreciative of the professionalism and expertise of our physicians, and the other health care professionals whom we encounter. Sometimes, however, it may be necessary to press for what we need. Herein applies the old adage "The squeaky wheel gets the grease". We certainly have a right to not be forgotten or ignored. If we find ourselves feeling that the machine is running completely without our input, then it's up to us to make the change. It may be time to "get squeaky". If we don't know what's going on in our treatment, then we bear some responsibility for addressing that dilemma. It may be that someone "should" keep us informed, but if that isn't happening, it is possible to remedy that situation. Rather than stewing over what some one or some system should be doing, we need to focus on finding out for ourselves. Have we asked? If we have asked, and received no response, then clearly that's the time to assert ourselves and to pursue our needs.

Of course, given the restrictions of our circumstances this may be more or less difficult to carry out. If we're injured on the job and are dealing with worker's compensation, we may feel trapped, and believe that we have to do what we're told and accept whatever is offered. In some ways this is true. But at the same time, it is often possible to get a second opinion; it is possible to sit down in the physician's office and get some answers. While being reasonable and prudent, we can be as involved in our treatment as possible. We can be proactive rather than reactive. We needn't feel victimized. This is not to say that we accept blame for our difficulties, just that we do what we can. We need to be sure that we are doing our part. Since there are so many things out of our control, it is vital we take responsibility for those actions over which we do have control. This will lead to feelings of confidence and adequacy, and the knowledge that we are in fact helping ourselves overcome adversity.

Mind and Body

As we begin to gather information, we also begin to understand the mind/body connection. As we are educated in how stress levels, emotional states, attitudes, and expectations affect our health, we get clues regarding what revisions will be necessary to optimize our health. We begin to understand that the statements "It's all in your head", or "It's just a medical problem", are artificial mental constructions.

It is easy for us to separate the concept of the body from that of the mind. The history of Western culture (at least for the past several hundred years) highlights this separation of body from mind. It began in the mid-1600's with the French philosopher Rene Descartes (often referred to as the Father of Modern philosophy), when he affirmed "Cogito, ergo sum"..."I think, therefore I am". He concluded that the possibility of conscious thought ("I think") scientifically demonstrated our existence ("therefore I am") as aware and mindful beings. This formed the basis of his assertion that the universe was composed of two discrete "substances", mind and matter (body).

This separation of mind from body and the consequent birth of the scientific method is probably the strength of Western medicine. The physician Andrew Weil proclaims that Western medicine is the worlds' best when it comes to acute medical care. If you need to go to the Emergency Room, there's probably no better place on the planet to go than the United States. He also states that the West (and the United States in particular) is less adept when it comes to treating chronic illness and pain. I agree. Eastern cultures have researched the realm of life-long health and its mirror image…chronic illness, injury and pain for several thousand years. Chinese Medicine in particular has had this focus for close to 5,000 years. Eastern medicine's knowledge base (until quite recently) was established from the "inside out", looking to the personal experience of mind and body for healing clues. Western medicine, on the other hand, has tended to take the route of finding such clues from dissecting a cadaver. The technical, scientific approach (Western) is distinguished from the intuitive, experiential approach (Eastern). The "scientific method" emphasizes test and retest, hypothesis and deduction. Intuition and any potential "subjective" opinions are systematically excluded from the final scientific conclusions.

And let me emphasize that this approach is not "bad". Clearly Descartes' method has been eminently beneficial (e.g. Man visits the moon and extends the life span of the planet's inhabitants). But while useful the scientific method is nonetheless only a utility, a tool and should not be confused with reality itself. When the professionals suggest we're imagining our problem, just because they can't see it, then the mental construct is no longer truly useful…it has become destructive. The *whole person* must be considered. This goes far beyond skin and bones.

Let me illustrate the mind/body connection. Many of us have had the experience of waking up on "the wrong side of the bed" after a bad night's sleep. Similarly, many of us have had the experience of having a hard time concentrating when we were in pain or ill. Or you may recall a time when you made an error in judgment as your thinking was affected by your physical state. The point I'm making, of course, is that our body affects our mental and emotional state. By contrast, consider your physical response if you were thinking to yourself "I'd like to wring so-and-so's neck!" or "Gee, I wonder what sort of shape I'll be in by the end of the day today?" Your heart rate and breathing-rate elevate, your muscles tense, your stomach knots up, and adrenaline starts coursing through your system. Mind affects body no less than body affects mind. We could even use the term "mind/body" or "body/mind" to invite and encourage a more inclusive perspective.

Nonetheless, we in the West are left with the dichotomy that separates our mind from our body. Under the circumstances, it is not surprising that we have a difficult time believing that things are "for real" if we don't have factual, objective data on which to base our conclusions and validate our experience. If we don't know the cause, if we don't know why we've got the symptoms, if we don't understand the mechanism or dynamic of the illness or pain, then we are often at a loss. Life feels just that much more uncertain, and an extra measure of anxiety is provoked. Whatever our convictions in this regard, we will benefit by being as informed as possible regarding the nature of our illness or injury.

Healthy Defiance

As we gain a mature understanding of the nature of our illness, pain, and injury, we can set realistic expectations for our daily activities and even for the long-term outcomes of our condition. Beyond the information remember to also trust your intuition and judgment. There's a fine balance between acceptance and a certain warrior-like defiance that keeps hope alive, and keeps us moving toward being as healthy as possible. Marc Ian Barasch, in *The* Healing Path, A Soul Approach to Illness, points to research done with terminally ill cancer patients who were defined by the health care providers as militant or resistant. He makes the point that those patients were often the ones who enjoyed miraculous remissions or significantly lengthened life spans. They trusted their own wisdom and challenged the status quo. This is not bitter denial and noncompliance, but rather life-affirming assertiveness. This approach demonstrates a healthy respect for *our* wisdom, as well as the wisdom of the experts.

Miraculous stories are, of course, the exception, but nonetheless, such things are possible. Our ability to find the balance between surrender and "the fight" leads us in the direction of healing. I propose that what will help us find that balance is our ability to clarify the healing responsibilities and capabilities of the medical, health care, and wellness community. The information we gather will then lend focus to our vision regarding our personal responsibilities in the healing journey. This will in turn clarify whether to surrender or fight, and what strategy will be most effective if we choose the fight. While there will most certainly be some "We really don't know" responses, we'll be wiser for it nonetheless. At least we asked. We can learn to cope with our given measure of uncertainty. So, let's ask once more, "It's up to who?"

Summary

- It is important that we understand as much as we can about our diagnosis and treatment. This enables us to most effectively participate in our treatment and to develop realistic expectations for our daily routines and plans.
- We must actively seek information from the health care community, books, the Internet, etc. Be creative in this search.
- Bring a list of questions and concerns. Take notes when you meet with health care providers.
- The separation between mind and body is an artificial mental construction. Their interrelation is the source of great opportunities for responsible selfcare.
- We must find the balance between acceptance and a healthy defiance that utilizes our intuition and wisdom to its best advantage. This energizes feelings of confidence and adequacy.

This book is INTERACTIVE…

Are you noticing that finally there is no one to blame and the ball is in your court?

To get access to more resources visit…

http://michaelgusac.ibi3g.com/MYBK5

PART TWO

The Management

WHAT'S SO FUNNY?

Overdoing It

MANY OF US have heard that laughter is good medicine. And probably most of us have, at one time or another tried to cheer somebody up by joking with him or her and getting them to laugh. We find that as they do so, it seems to help them get their mind off their troubles. This works particularly well when it comes to children, as we are able to distract them from their upset and redirect their focus, often to the point of their actually forgetting about what it was that upset them. When chronic illness or injury persistently haunts us, however, it's not so easy to forget. In fact, we may even find ourselves resentful when someone tries to cheer us up. It's as if we were being told that we were wrong to have our feelings, that we were wrong to be upset. The underlying message seems to be "Stop feeling that way". We might even the experienced of feeling a great deal of anger toward the person who encouraged us to "put on a happy face", or "snap out of it".

Humor can be ill timed and inappropriate. Indiscriminately joking about anything and everything will not contribute to our recovery.

Humor is then being used in the extreme as an escape. Constantly joking about our pain to the point where we never emotionally experience it (because the laughter becomes a method to *avoid* and *deny* the pain) will, in the long run, be counterproductive. We will inevitably be overwhelmed by the feelings that we use our humor to ameliorate. Occasionally, I see someone making this mistake, but frankly, over doing it with laughter is rarely a problem in the arena of pain and illness. More often, the tendency is to become bitter and morbid, with a cynical outlook that consistently anticipates disaster.

When I speak of humor, what interests me most is the attitude that it engenders. A sense of humor regarding ones injury seems to allows us to temporarily detach and distance ourselves from the pain of our illness or injury. It is that detachment, that ability to objectively observe ourselves and our situation that offers up opportunities for healing and recovery. But before I wax philosophical, let's explore for a moment the physiological aspects of laughter.

Laughter and the Body

It has been observed that we use a significantly greater number of facial muscles to generate a frown than a smile. This suggests that smiling requires less energy, is more relaxing, and less tension producing than frowning. The frown both generates and reflects the stress and tension we feel. There is research that suggests that neuro-chemicals (substances that transmit nerve impulses) such as the endorphins (morphinelike substances naturally produced in our body) are generated when we laugh. This suggests that our physical sensitivity to pain can be reduced, as we are able to laugh.

There is a book written by Norman Cousins recounting his recovery from ankylosing spondylitis (a debilitating and excruciatingly painful bone disease) wherein he affirms that the use of humor provided the relief that all medical treatments had failed to provide. He watched comedy movies (e.g. movies by Charlie Chaplin and the

Marx Brothers) for hours at a time, on a daily basis, and cultivated humor throughout every aspect of his daily routine. His contention was that it revitalized his healing and recuperative abilities. And, in fact, blood tests validated the presence of chemical substances related to pain relief, and to an improvement in his condition one to two hours after his laughter therapy. He believes that this was the primary cause of his recovery. While he was not permanently "cured", he was able to resume his work as editor of a prominent magazine.

We may not want to take it to that extreme as we consider the virtues of humor; nonetheless, it certainly seems to be worth our attention. Both physiologically and biochemically, the benefits to be derived from laughter are potentially numerous and far-reaching. We are highlighting the potential for mood elevation, decreased sensitivity to pain, efficient use of the musculature of the face and hands, and efficient utilization of the body's healing capabilities, i.e., the enhancement of our immune system.

Humor and Detachment

Let us now explore what type of attitude it takes to develop and maintain a sense of humor in the challenging circumstances of chronic illness and injury.

It is clear to me that one of the great values of laughter is that it helps us step back more objectively and observe our circumstances. It also helps us avoid the pitfalls of taking our problems and ourselves too seriously. If we take them too seriously, as their importance is exaggerated and they become overwhelming, we become embittered and enmeshed in a web of self-pity. We lose sight of the fact that we are not alone. As that happens, we become increasingly isolated and obsessed with our problems in a way that overshadows the rest of our daily experience and awareness. These can be powerful and often intense emotions, which require strong medicine to remedy. Very often humor is the best prescription available.

It is vital that we are able to laugh at ourselves, and that we practice this attitude with sufficient frequency to keep us reminded of the fact that as bad as we've got it, there is much for which we can be grateful. As we are able to laugh at ourselves, our circumstances and the absurd unfairness of it all, we are less caught up with ourselves. Pride and selfpity will interfere less in our day.

Here's an example of chronic illness humor (is this where the term "sick" humor came from?). My cousin recounted to me a Christmas party for Crohn's patients where Santa passed out gifts such as: Christmas toilet paper, preparation-H, Maalox tablets, and other bowel-related products. She went on to relate that some of the Crohn's patients laughed so hard she thought they "might blow an artery".

I'm not sure which comes first, the detachment or the laughter, the humor or the objectivity. It certainly seems to require objectivity in order to forego taking ourselves too seriously. As we are able to laugh at ourselves, we become more detached. If I am able to tell a story on myself, to recount an event that I find humorous related to my difficulties, I also find that sharing this with others helps me maintain my equilibrium, a balanced perspective on my difficulties. This does not minimize the challenges, but it can diminish their power and impact on us.

Early in my adjustment to my kidney problem, my initial reactions were those of, guilt, anxiety, and frustration. In contrast, as I was coping with my nerve illness, I was able to tell stories on myself, to laugh at some of my limitations, and to take the role of observer regarding other problems as well. To illustrate, as my nerve illness progressed, and I became weaker and number, there was an occasion where I was unable to get my shoe on the foot that was most affected by the symptoms of numbness and tingling. Try as I might I could not get that shoe on. I put on thinner, sheerer socks, but to no avail. I assumed that the numbness indicated that my foot was swelling and in fact larger than it had previously been. Finally, I put on another pair of shoes (loose fitting loafers), and this worked quite nicely…. it was the same scenario the following day. On the third day, it occurred to me to look in my shoe. As I did, I discovered that there was a sock stuffed in my shoe!

I often recount this episode to groups that I facilitate. When this initially happened, I shared it with my co-workers in the outpatient clinic where I worked at the time with a sense of amusement regarding how hyper-vigilant I had become. I had become so governed by my assumptions about the numbness, that it did not even occur to me to do what would normally have been my first response! Normally, if I can't get my foot in my shoe, I would assume there must be something in it. While I may have had a few good reasons to get a bit sidetracked the point is if we take our illness or injury too seriously, we can distort our experience and limit our options and our creative intelligence. My response to my Guillain-Barre' included an ability to view this incident as something that was laughable, and to objectively see myself as someone who was overwhelmed by his preoccupation with his illness. And perhaps the most valuable part of this incident was that I was able to share it with others without embarrassment, guilt, or shame because I wasn't taking my difficulties or myself too seriously.

The ability to "lighten up" a bit in the midst of challenges and even tragedy can be a great relief, as it decreases the tension levels that can so easily exhaust us. It's as if we had dropped the sand ballast from a hot air balloon, and floated skyward to enjoy the panoramic vistas of a detached and more complete perspective. Humor can then create an awareness of the positive, hopeful aspects of our daily experience. It is much easier to feel grateful and encouraged when we actively cultivate our sense of humor in a way that allows us to step back and observe the lives of others, as well as our own life. We may discover that in this attitude rest the seeds of happiness and opportunities for decreasing the impact of our pain and illness. Our symptoms can abate to some degree. The attitude is: "Don't take it *too* seriously." Detach. Observe. Enjoy!

Summary

- Humor can be overdone. It then becomes an escape.
- Laughter can provide physiological pain relief.
- Humor helps us to establish and maintain an objective outlook regarding our difficulties.
- Cultivate the ability to laugh at yourself. Learn to occasionally "lighten up" and be less serious about your situation.

This book is INTERACTIVE...

When you are overwhelmed by the pain, laughter can provide needed perspective.

To get access to more resources visit...

http://michaelgusac.odgi.net/MYBK6

IF YOU "FEEL" LIKE DOING IT...DON'T!

Depression as Illness

IT REALLY DOESN'T require any detailed description of our circumstances to help us understand the situations and experiences that contribute to feeling depressed. Our loss can be profound. We may lose our *livelihood*. We can lose our *independence,* as we may have to begin asking for help for the first time in our lives, or have to depend on insurance, spouse, or family for income. We may lose our sense of *personal identity*, our sense of Self, as our capabilities become more limited. We may lose our *confidence* in our judgement or overall competence. The losses can extend to *literally every* area of our lives. Chronic injury, pain, and illness have a power and pervasiveness that defies description.

Depression is a curious thing. The ways in which we think, and the things we are naturally inclined to do, or not do, are precisely the ones that will tend to maintain our depression. When we're depressed, for example, we tend to notice what's going wrong...the proverbial glass that's half empty vs. the one that's half full. Certainly that can be quite depressing. We feel like doing absolutely nothing when we're depressed. This too will tend to keep us depressed. But before we go into a great deal of detail in this itemization, let's consider just what I mean when I say we're depressed.

There is a difference between being "sad" and being "depressed". Depression is more powerful and pervasive than sadness. In fact we have learned that depression is actually a medical illness for which medication can often provide relief, no less than we might use insulin if we were diabetic. The research suggests that our brains do not produce certain chemicals in the proper proportions when we're depressed, and that this imbalance affects our ability to maintain emotional equilibrium. As a consequence, depression affects us physically, as well as emotionally. Here's a list of symptoms that can indicate depression:

1. Low energy levels: fatigue
2. Sleep disruption—too much or too little sleep
3. Appetite disruption—too much or too little eating
4. Irritability
5. Poor concentration—problems with short term memory
6. Tearfulness
7. Feelings of hopelessness
8. Feeling helpless or powerless
9. Indecisiveness
10. Death looks like a means of attaining peace; suicide may be contemplated

This list is fairly comprehensive, but not exhaustive. The symptoms are thought to indicate depression as a clinical illness if we've experienced them consistently for a period of two weeks. The first three on the list are clearly physical manifestations. The next three are combine body and mind. And the last four symptoms are emotional and spiritual in expression. Let's use the list to differentiate sad from depressed.

When we're sad, we have reasons for our tears. But when we're depressed, tears come "out of the blue" often for no apparent reason. Concentration is not a big problem when we're sad. Weight loss or gain is not a concern when we're sad. Memory is usually fairly intact when we're sad. Suicide is certainly not an issue with sadness. When we're only getting two to four hours of sleep; when we're having problems with weight gain and loss; when deciding on what to eat at the restaurant or McDonalds is a major issue, then we're probably depressed. When we're tearful for no particular reason; when we can't remember why we are standing at the door to our room; when we angrily overreact to someone tipping over the saltshaker, then we may be depressed. I'm referring to patterns of reacting and behaving over a period of time— not just an isolated incident.

Now, you may be thinking that chronic pain or illness could explain many of these symptoms. You fox! That is absolutely true. However, the intensity of the symptoms is not likely to be as great, or to be as persistent. But teasing this out is not easy. It is often a bit of both vs. either/or (either pain or depression being attributed as the causal factor). Nonetheless, depression is a force with which we must deal. It's difficult to effect a healthy adjustment to a chronic condition when we're feeling doomed! So what do we do?

Challenging Our Depression

Whatever we feel like doing when we're depressed; we need to do just the opposite! If we feel like avoiding the world, isolating ourselves, and talking to nobody, we need to create an opportunity to be with friends or family. When we feel like sleeping the day away, we need to get out of bed and take on a project. When we don't feel like engaging in that hobby that "used to" interest us, we need to do it anyway (within the limits of our abilities of course). If we don't feel like eating anything today, we need to eat despite our lack of appetite. If taking that walk around the block is the last thing in the world we want to do today, then we can make it the *first*. If everything seems to be the same, then we can start looking for differences—in our symptoms, in situations, and in others. Now when it comes to looking for "differences", depressed thinking will definitely present us with a challenge. It's easy to notice whatever seems the *same* when we are depressed. All-or-nothing, either/or, black-or-white thinking, is the depressed order of the day. To effectively challenge this depressive thinking inclination let me suggest a strategy for beginning to notice differences in our symptoms. This is the best way to establish hope for a brighter day with some prospect for again feeling joy and happiness.

We can evaluate our depressive symptoms using these three criteria: (a) frequency (b) duration and (c) intensity. Take sleep for example. If asked, we could accurately report that our sleep is "still pretty bad". Now, while this might be true, it may also be true that we slept four hours instead of two hours (duration). While inadequate, four hours is certainly an improvement over two. The quality of our sleep could be more valuable than the actual length of time for which we slept. Perhaps our sleep, while only for two hours, was more restful (intensity). We may have observed that while we slept poorly five days out of the week, there were two nights when our sleep was almost back to normal (frequency). We actually had two good nights. So as we practice looking for differences, we can ask "How often?" "How long?" and "How much?"

Let me offer one other example to illustrate how we might apply these criteria to our symptoms. Let's consider anger for a moment. *Frequency*: How often do you get upset and angry? Even if the intensity and length of time that you are angry were no different, getting angry once a day vs. hourly *would* be different. Or perhaps the incidence of your anger shifts from daily to once a week. Now that would be a noticeable difference! Wouldn't it? *Duration*: If you calm down quicker, are not upset for as long, that counts as a difference, as progress. *Intensity*: If you don't get as angry (even if it happens as often *and* for as long), then this can be considered progress.

The most obvious and desirable progress would, of course, take place on all three fronts. But in the early stages of recovery from depression, it's important to distinguish every aspect of change no matter how small. This will help us break the habit of depressive thinking. And it can become a habit in a very short period of time. Since this habit can be hard to break, the differences should be considered that much more significant. All change is significant under these circumstances. There are no small, insignificant changes.

Roadblocks

Let's consider a few typical roadblocks to resolving the depression with which we may be struggling. The thought may occur "I don't feel like getting out of bed." Well consider this. Did you ever have the experience of telling yourself "I don't feel like going to work today" while you were putting the keys in the ignition of your car? Most of us know how to do what we don't feel like doing. It's a matter of priorities. Obviously financial survival is high on everyone's priority list. That's why we sometimes drive to work regardless of our preference. Now, in dealing with our injury/illness, it's a matter of placing self-care and health high enough on our priority list so that "I don't feel like it" is no longer sufficient reason to refuse to do what would further our recovery from our depression.

Another thought that tends to interfere is "I just don't have the time". We discover that we can get quite creative if we decide the project is sufficiently important. Then it will get done. For instance, we may have told ourselves when we felt the need to take a break from a project, that we couldn't *afford* the time it took to do so. The break seemed to take away from the time required for the projects' completion. Well, when we're depressed (as well as with other aspects of our injury/illness), we can't afford to *not* take the steps required to elevate our mood, and ease our emotional pain.

An Initial Plan

Let's assume that we've decided we are, in fact, depressed, and that we've gotten beyond these few roadblocks. Here's a brief plan incorporating the attitudes and information we've discussed.

- *Daily Walk*—Set an initial goal of walking four out of seven days per week. Five minutes a day is fine for a start. Twenty or thirty minutes would, of course, be better, but consistency is what is most important. Better to walk a little bit every day than an hour twice a week.
- *Look for differences*—This will help challenge and reorganize depressive thinking patterns. Pay attention primarily to the list of symptoms of depression. And apply the criteria of frequency, duration, and intensity as you so. Think FDI – not FBI (Federal Bureau of Investigation) mind you, but FDI, using the distinction between D and B-and the association with FBI for the purpose of helping you keep the criteria in mind.
- *Do One Good Thing For Yourself Each Day*—It's important to take responsibility for meeting our emotional and spiritual needs…even if we don't feel like it… perhaps especially if we don't feel like it. This doesn't have to be anything particularly dramatic. Whatever seems like a spiritual treat counts. Listening to some music, talking to a friend, a hot soak in the tub, or reading something spiritually uplifting could serve this purpose.

Our intention to nourish our spirit is what counts… regardless of the specific activity.

- *Spend Time with Others*—Don't isolate yourself. You may find that socializing makes you feel a bit anxious and uncomfortable. Do it anyway. Isolation leads to a preoccupation with our problem, which leads to self-pity. Self-pity will simply exacerbate the depression.

- *Seek Medical Attention If Necessary*—If the symptoms of depression as distinguished from sadness persist for more than a few weeks consult your family physician. He or she may want to refer you to counseling, or to begin you on a trial of anti-depressant medication. Remember that depression is an illness, and may require some medication to re-establish the normal biochemical balance so that the coping tools we utilize will be most effective.

As you consider whether to initiate this plan, for it's quite possible that you won't *feel* like following through with it just fake it for a bit. It may contradict your natural inclinations at this point, but you need to keep in mind that depressed thinking tends to be distorted. We tend to notice what reinforces our mood. Bad news seems like the only news in town. Initiate this plan for two to four weeks. Then evaluate once more.

Summary

- We have experienced losses in many areas of our life as a consequence of our injury/illness. The effects are pervasive and powerful.

- Depression is a medical illness. As such it may require medication as part of the remedy. Depression is not the same thing as sadness. It affects us on a physical as well as a spiritual/emotional level.

- We need to challenge our natural inclinations when we are depressed. That which we are inclined to think or do will tend to keep us depressed.

- Look for differences in your symptoms, and in your surroundings. There are certain criteria that can help us make these distinctions. Look for changes in the frequency, duration, and intensity levels of your symptoms.

- Be aware of the potential roadblocks that may interfere with your most effective recovery. We can institute a basic plan, which will challenge the typical features of depression, and create the best opportunity for regaining equilibrium.

This book is INTERACTIVE…

Depression can be draining, but your feelings don't have to make your decisions for you.

You can take control by visiting…

http://michaelgusac.ibi3g.com/MYBK7

IT JUST ISN'T WORTH IT

Justified Anger

MANY OF US have learned over time that anger is unacceptable. It has been made clear to us that it would be wiser to keep it to ourselves. There are to be no demonstrations of the fact that we are upset. The underlying message is "If you don't have anything good to say, then don't say anything at all." The only acceptable expressions are positive, cheerful, compliant ones. We are left with that age-old strategy of keeping it to ourselves and suppressing that nasty old anger. Well, that may make life comfortable for those around us, but it tends to be a counterproductive, if not destructive strategy for the person invoking it. This is what is known as "suppressing" feelings. And, if the feelings become buried so deep that they are typically beyond our conscious ability to recall, then we call these feelings "repressed." Feelings become more difficult to manage if we're not even aware that they exist.

Heaven knows we've got reasons to be upset. There are numerous things that can trigger our anger. People can be unsympathetic toward us when they are ignorant of the limitations chronic illness and injury pose. If we're not obviously missing a body part, then people react as if it's "All in your head", that we are imagining this illness, this pain, and this limitation. Or worse yet people react as if we're "faking it"; pretending that a problem exists when it really does not or that the problem is worse that it really is. It can be annoying, if not enraging; to feel misunderstood, to feel discounted. And even those who live with us, in their own denial and frustration, may at times believe we're making things worse than they really are.

As we experience a long list of losses relative to the chronic nature of our problem, one of our natural reactions to such loss is anger. It makes us angry when we can't do what we once could, particularly if, by comparison with our past abilities, it's something "simple" like washing the dishes or mowing the lawn. We become angry, if we can't earn the salary we once could. When we feel abandoned by friends and family, anger is a typical response to the pain of that loss. We find ourselves reacting angrily to the unending parade of medical appointments and procedures we have to endure. It all gets abysmally tiresome, often exhausting, and at times infuriating.

Since we have good reasons to be angry, it is important that we give ourselves permission to feel our anger so that we do not stuff it, ignore it, or try to pretend it away. This avoidance is rarely an effective strategy. We often discover that we're only postponing its inevitable outburst and eruption. We must acknowledge our anger, and find a way to constructively utilize it. A time out can be helpful, but it is then important to return to the incident or issue that triggered our reaction.

The Consequences of Ignoring Anger

While an angry outburst may be upsetting and destructive, it is rarely as destructive as what may come from harboring the anger over an extended period of time. Resentment and bitterness are powerful, pervasive, and potentially debilitating emotions. The terms resentment and bitterness refer to the kind of anger that creates an open wound that refuses to heal. This wound affects us spiritually in a way that transforms our personality, and makes not only our life, but also the lives of those around us a miserable experience. We become "hard to live with". We are constantly looking for a fight. Our very presence seems to have the ability to infect others with our venom, and joy, happiness, and satisfaction are quickly sucked right out of our lives.

The clients with whom I work who have the hardest time adjusting to the chronicity of their illness or injury are those who are choking on a steady diet of anger. It can suffocate them before they are even aware it's a problem. Anger's power and subtlety is imposing. Early on in the process of suppressing or "stuffing" anger, we're irritable more often than not. Then one day we abruptly discover that we are easily enraged by the most ridiculous, inconsequential minutia. "Don't you look at me that way!" we scream. Spilling the saltshaker is enough to trigger a temper tantrum.

We become suspicious and mistrustful. We expect the worst, and our attitude and behavior often create circumstances where our expectations are met and the worst actually does come to pass. Regardless of how justified we may be in our reactions to our difficulties, there comes a point at which we are wallowing in self-pity and punishing whoever is within striking distance. We are then taking advantage of the people who love and care about us, for they cannot escape our wrath unless they choose separation or divorce. Our spouses may not physically leave us because they love us. Our children have no choice but to endure our mood. However, they will all most certainly have to begin to emotionally separate themselves from us in order to survive. And whether or not we have children and spouses, friends and other family members will begin to limit their contact with us. Often the truth is not that others abandon us, but rather that we drive them away. Their lack of compassion and empathy is quite understandable.

Not only does it affect our mood and behavior, but our pent-up anger can also affect our prospects for physical recovery. We are less likely to take care of ourselves out of our conviction that it won't do any good anyway. We convince ourselves that it's just a waste of our time. We are less likely to ask for what we need, because we assume that others will not be responsive. A plethora of stress related problems could begin to emerge. Our pain levels increase. We become susceptible to colds and other illnesses. We begin to get headaches.

It Just Isn't Worth It

We may begin to realize over time (and sometimes, unfortunately, we're talking about years) that holding on to our anger is an exhausting enterprise that ironically tends to hurt us and those we cherish more than it does any real or imagined transgressor. The people with whom we are upset often don't care whether we're angry with them, and are not even aware that we *are* angry with them. Just soaking in the anger produces few effects beyond making *us* miserable. Bitterness is a good word for this lingering, boiling emotion, for it certainly leaves a bad taste in one's mouth.

At this point we need to make a decision, or at least ask ourselves a question regarding our priorities. Is it more important for us to be happy, or is it more important to be "Right?" While we may be justified in our righteous indignation, what benefit is really to be had? Over time, we conclude that our happiness and the happiness of those we love is more important than being "right". We begin to say to ourselves "It just isn't worth it", because we understand that feelings of resentment and bitterness are a colossal waste of energy and time. No good comes of it, and much harm will be done. We choose an attitude that keeps the intensity of our feelings manageable.

We also realize that it isn't worth it because there are limits to what we can control. We have little or no control over someone's negative attitude toward us (often energized by their ignorance of the restrictions imposed on us by our illness or injury). Neither do we have final control over how others choose to behave toward us. We can't "make" them behave as we wish. We have limited control over the injustices of life in general, or the insurance or medical "systems" in particular.

There really is nothing we can do about some of these inequities, and we will feel better if we let go of the subsequent feelings of rage and indignation they engender regardless of our justification for having them. We conclude that to live in anger over things we cannot change or control is a project in which we are no longer willing to engage. Again we realize it's a waste of our time and energy. It's important to acknowledge that we are angry but, having done so, we can then explore how to bring the turmoil to some sort of resolution. We need to harness and utilize this anger.

Listening to Anger

Well, what precisely is it in anger that we can utilize? We can harness the energy that anger mobilizes to take concrete action appropriate to the circumstances. Our anger may be telling us that we have been injured emotionally or spiritually and need to take measures to heal the wound. For instance, if I have been humiliated and my feelings are hurt, I may benefit by confronting the person or situation without delay…no time for resentments to grow. If confrontation does not fit the circumstances, then a resolution to avoid similar injuries in the future may be prudent. Our anger may tell us that we have been attacked and need to protect ourselves. A good example is encountering an employer that is refusing to honor his/her obligations to provide benefits after we've been injured on the job. Or perhaps we're encountering resistance from worker's compensation in providing timely treatment. Then our anger could motivate us to secure legal counsel to protect our rights. Our anger would be functioning in a constructive manner…no festering resentment here either.

Anger may be telling us that our needs are not being met… our emotional needs for security and affection, spiritual needs for faith and hope, or physical needs for food and shelter would all be examples. Here we can utilize our anger by assertively taking personal responsibility for meeting our needs, as opposed to waiting for someone else to meet them and then feeling victimized if they don't. Of course, we are not self sufficient, but I'm emphasizing that anger can engage productive action.

Bitterness and resentment can also be put to use in the service of our health and well-being. It is resentment that can teach us the consequences of being chronically angry. And as we learn this lesson, as we receive this message, we can then choose a different emotional and behavioral course. While the chronic nature of our injury/illness may be largely out of our control, resolving chronic emotional distress is an area over which we can exert a great deal of influence. We can clarify for ourselves the limits of our control, and realize that *our* thoughts and behaviors are things over which we finally *do* have some control and for which *we* bear responsibility.

We can begin to repeat to ourselves the following series of statements: "There's just nothing I can do about this", "I need to let it go", "It just isn't worth it", "It's out of my control", "My health is more important than…." Here we have a combination of interrelated thoughts and attitudes that can energize a perspective that will shatter the seeming impenetrability of bitterness and resentment. Such selfstatements can diminish the intensity of these feelings, and eventually resolve most of them. These persistent feelings of anger that extend over the days, months, and years of our experience with our illness or injury can come to an end. Forgiveness begins as we choose to heal ourselves rather than punishing others.

We experience a new set of priorities that give us a much-welcomed tranquility. If it's not *worth* storing anger on a chronic basis, then what *is* worthwhile? We must find our own answers to this question, but I suspect we will conclude that our energy is better spent enjoying our friends and family, and the other priceless blessings that can uplift and enrich our lives. Better to savor good company, a breathtaking sunset, or a good meal than to fret over what "should be" but often isn't. Better to take time to heal spiritually, as well as emotionally and physically.

Caution! Roadblocks Ahead!

Let me alert you to a couple of potential obstructions to adopting this willingness to let go of resentment and bitterness. Many of us who really struggle with our anger come to believe that if we let go of the anger, there will be nothing left. We've spent so much time with our anger that it seems as if it's the only thing that is motivating us and keeping us from being engulfed by a state of frozen immobility. It has almost become a familiar and cherished friend. Anger may be energizing in the short term, but if we are chronically angry it begins to drain us as we find fatalism and depression beginning to drain our reserves. At this point, anger (which has now become resentment) limits rather than enhances our productivity. We learn however, that rather than being immobilized, we actually discover newfound energy reserves as we choose to take action to resolve the anger.

We also often come to believe that if we resolve our anger that this would be equivalent to saying "It's OK", and letting someone, or something off the hook. We think that if we let go of our anger, then we have to "forget it". Well, we are not required to forget any injustice that has been done. It is not necessary to say "It's OK." What *is* necessary is that we heal our wounds. I often challenge my clients to consider the possibility that the best revenge is to not simply survive when wronged, but to *thrive*. Perhaps this is a variation on the classic parental advice to ignore the bully who taunts us…just act as if we didn't hear them and go on about our daily business of growth and learning.

One other pitfall that may interfere with our ability to take on the "It's not worth it!" attitude is the specter of pride. Pride, in itself, is not a bad thing; it can work well for us. Pride can motivate us to achieve; it can contribute to our sense of worth and accomplishment. It can also lock us into a stubborn, destructive frame of mind; where we won't concede that we're not as strong as we thought we were or would like to be. And it can be quite a challenge to admit that we cannot do what we once could. This is particularly applicable when others continue to expect that we meet the performance standards that applied prior to our difficulties.

We are confronted with the paradox that our strength can become our weakness; that the way in which pride functions to motivate us toward excellence, now becomes an immobilizing prison. It is once again a question of balance. To utilize our pride to keep hope alive and pursue our recovery with a certain vengeance is the stuff of which stories of miraculous healing are made. But, at the same time, we must temper this defiance and ferocity with humility and an awareness of our humanity. To make a mistake doesn't mean we are "failures". We can be in need of help without being "weaklings". We can choose to relinquish our anger while maintaining our sense of self worth and pride. This is pride well placed…to put away the bitterness and claim the satisfaction that comes from a job well done. The job being the work of choosing to leave the past where it belongs, to enjoy the precious present moment, and to look ahead to a life of possibility and promise.

Summary

- We have many good reasons to be angry and upset. Our anger is justified.
- Bitterness and resentment are the chronic forms of anger.
- The consequences of unresolved anger are destructive and pervasive.
- We tend to suffer far more than the object toward which our anger is directed.
- Being angry about unchangeable realities is a waste of precious energy…energy that is better directed toward coping and healing.
- Anger should be utilized rather than extinguished.
- Awareness of potential roadblocks to resolving our anger will speed the healing process.

This book is INTERACTIVE…

You have so many legitimate reasons to be angry. But standing on that principle can drain the life out of you. To get access to more resources that can expand your coping options visit…

http://michaelgusac.odgi.net/MYBK8

THE LESS CONTROL WE NEED THE MORE CONTROL WE'LL HAVE

Fear and Uncertainty

"FEAR IS THE Mind Killer." This is one of the repeating themes in the science fiction novel *DUNE* by Frank Herbert. This statement is one of the foundations of the mystical religious order in his book. So what does that have to do with chronic illness and pain? The power of fear to limit our creativity and restrict our flexibility cannot be overstated. Fear shows up in many forms and with various degrees of intensity. We may call it "anxiety". We may call it "worry". We may call it "nervous tension". It may look like anger. And it may feel like terror. All of these variations, I believe, are related to our encounter with one of the harshest and, at the same time, most liberating realities of the human condition. I am referring to the fact that the amount of control we have over our circumstances, other peoples reactions, and life in general is far more limited than most of us are willing to admit or even consider. As we encounter "the Unknown" and its attendant uncertainty, fear is a typical reaction.

We may only be dimly aware of our fear. Don't underestimate its power or pervasiveness.

What does the future hold? What will others think? Will we get better? Will our condition get worse? How long do we have to live? Where will the money come from (for the bills…for present or future treatment)? Is this the right treatment approach? Is this the right doctor? Sound familiar? It does to many of us. And as we ask ourselves these questions, fear is the common reaction…as is our denial and avoidance of that fear. Life typically seems predictable and "normal". Most of us are able to live (and often prefer to live) under the illusion that the rules that apply today will also apply tomorrow. None of us can really afford to spend our time looking over our shoulders wondering what disaster may befall us (denial does have its place). We believe the sun will rise every morning, and that we will make it home intact each day as we return from our place of business. We assume that when we arrive home, comfort and security will be waiting. We look at one side of a building and assume that the other side is there, even though we cannot actually see it.

Consider our illness or injury. In the acute stages, the rules still seem to apply. But as the problem becomes "chronic" (defined as 'lasting longer than three months'), life's certainties, the sympathy and understanding of others, and perhaps even our financial situation, all begin to erode. What worked well for so long now begins to work against us. The illusion of complete control vanishes.

Isolation

Some of us, as we adjust to the inescapable uncertainties of our illness, pain, or injury, choose to protect ourselves by isolating ourselves. If we stay at home, the world seems much safer. We don't have to wonder about whether we're going to be able to follow through with that social activity we scheduled. We don't have to tolerate the embarrassment and shame we may feel due to being limited, feeling handicapped, even "crippled", if there's no one else to see it. There's nobody asking us questions about our problems. There are no requirements or demands. Life seems much safer, and it is definitely more predictable.

This strategy for gaining some sense of control in an "out of control" situation will backfire however if we let it become a pattern. Our retreat becomes our prison. We no longer feel competent to negotiate normal social situations and, before we know it, we're refusing to answer the door or the phone when it rings. We begin to avoid events where we anticipate any sort of demand on us to interact with other people.

As a consequence, we begin to feel trapped, suffocated, and even claustrophobic. It's not unusual, at this point, for us to begin feeling nervous while driving, crossing a bridge, riding in an elevator, or being in a room without windows. We fear we may crash off the bridge into the water. We anticipate the elevator cable snapping as we plummet to our death. We can actually feel the walls closing in on us. All of these situations remind us of the possibility that something could happen which will be out of our control.

On the other extreme, the world looms too large when we feel insecure and vulnerable and there is nothing but uncertainty and unknowns. This feels equally threatening and forbidding. However, we discover in the adjustment to our injury/illness that avoidance is the wrong remedy. It provides a temporary, but false sense of security. Avoidance will multiply rather than reduce the problems we're experiencing. A pattern of running away from whatever it is that makes us uncomfortable is a project that is doomed to failure. As we attempt to escape our fear, we discover that it runs just as fast as we can. Whenever we stop running and look around, we discover that it's still with us. If we don't face our discomfort and fear, it will come to control us, and we will discover that fear and avoidance are shaping our behavior.

It is well documented that if we have a fearful or phobic reaction to any particular environmental stimulus, that, eventually, it takes less and less to trigger the same reaction. Initially we're afraid of a snake, and before we know it, the *word* "snake" can throw us into a tailspin. And more in keeping with our theme consider that just anticipating the pain of a particular diagnostic or treatment procedure, just seeing it scheduled on the calendar could be the stimulus sufficient to actually trigger a panic episode. And when I say panic, I mean a full-blown physical reaction sufficiently intense to send us to the hospital emergency room scared to death that we're having a heart attack. This is a physical reaction complete with chest pain, pounding heart, shortness of breath, and a feeling of impending doom (to name but a few of the panic symptoms). This is the extreme, but it can and *does* happen…and to some of my "strongest" clients.

To master our fear requires that we spend time with it because escape and avoidance certainly don't work…at least not in the larger view. We must also challenge the thoughts which fear can energize. We must challenge the catastrophic thoughts that exaggerate any uncertain outcome into an expected disaster. We must challenge the belief that avoidance provides long-term relief. Obviously avoidance (often known as the "easy way out") usually provides immediate relief. The point is that the relief doesn't last, the problem doesn't magically evaporate, and our reactions become progressively worse. We must stop running, avoiding, and isolating ourselves from our fear and pain.

Letting Go Daily

What we discover over time is that living in the present moment and approaching the day with flexibility is what allows us the greatest degree of security and serenity. As the day begins we never quite know how we are going to feel or how the day is going to turn out. As we accept this *fact* (and I emphasize the word "fact"), we notice that we feel less anxious and fearful. We are calmer and better able to adapt to varying circumstances. We are able to let go of our need to control the outcomes of circumstances. We also stop trying to control other people and "make" them think or act as we wish.

Oddly enough, as we relinquish control and loosen our grip on life we experience a greater sense of control. We feel empowered in our newfound ability to manage our reaction to the unpredictable and unknown aspects of our pain, injury, or illness. This ability stems from an attitude of "watchfulness", of almost idle curiosity. We limit our assumptions about how the day will turn out, and creatively respond to the requirements of each event as it occurs.

One of the best ways I've found to begin to let go of our need to control events and others is to cultivate the faith that things will work out in the long run regardless of whether they work out the way we would wish in the short term. We can look back on our experience to those times when we thought an event was a "misfortune." However, further down the line in the long view, that misfortune turned out to be "fortunate"; it "worked out for the best after all." This remembrance can help us develop such belief, such faith. And faith is probably a better term, since it's meaning also allows for the presence of doubt. *Belief* as a concept implies that there is *complete* certainty. With *faith* we don't have to be totally convinced that things will "work out". Faith makes "letting go" and relaxing into the day's circumstances far more feasible.

Worry

While we may have interrupted the patterns of isolation and avoidance, there will probably be times when our faith will fail us and we will begin worrying excessively. I consider worry to be an indirect attempt at regulation and control of life's circumstances and outcomes. When we worry, we play an elaborate chess game, anticipating moves and counter-moves, as we attempt to plan a strategy to address each possible eventuality. "If this happens, what will I do?"

we ask ourselves. "And if that happens, how will it turn out?" we wonder. Aren't we really trying to somehow control the outcome, to insure that things will work out the way we want?

The futility of worry becomes obvious when we fret over something for days, anticipating how we might deal with a certain occurrence, and then it never comes to pass. Whatever we anticipated, it didn't even happen. We are then left thinking "What a waste of time! I spent all that time worrying about nothing!"

What does worry actually accomplish? Usually very little, and certainly for the amount of time and energy we invest in worrying, we're not getting a good return on our investment. A client once gave me a placard with the inscription: *Worry is like a rocking chair. There's lots of movement, but we never get anywhere.* I'm reminded of the hamster feverishly running in the wheel in its cage…we get just about as far. But, chances are, the hamster has a good deal more fun.

Worry is repeatedly thinking and rethinking, anticipating and again anticipating, in a way that consumes our energy, attention, and concentration. We can actually worry ourselves sick. Tension levels increase. Pain levels increase. We suffer from headaches, stomachaches, diarrhea, ulcers, and a long list of other symptoms. If this happens with any regularity, we will conclude that here, as with resentment, it just isn't "worth it". Yet despite this conclusion we may not be able to stop worrying.

Worry Limiting Strategies

If you just can't stop worrying, you might want to try some of the following strategies:

1. Choose to *compartmentalize* worry. This involves setting aside a certain time of day for worrying. Pretend that the problem is not that you are worrying too much, but that

you are not worrying *properly*. Very often our worry is in the background as we go about the days activities, but we never take it to its final conclusion (e.g. considering the worst case scenario). We never truly confront our bottom-line fears or finally decide on what we are to do. Consequently, what we need to do is sit down with our concerns and take them from beginning to end, "burn it out", and then let it go. Then what you tell yourself during the day is "I'm not going to worry about that now; I'll think about that this evening at 6:30." Set aside a day, an hour, a half hour, ten minutes…whatever it takes and whenever you prefer. You might even be surprised to find that you're unable to worry when the allotted time arrives. When your worry time is over, do something else and get your mind off those concerns.

2. If your worries disrupt your sleep, one helpful strategy is to write your concerns down on paper. This helps objectify the thoughts; it gets them "out there". It also helps slow them down. And often, you will gain new insight into the problem.

3. If we are spiritually oriented, we could try using a "God Bag". This involves getting a paper bag, or perhaps a small trashcan, and literally labeling it the "God Bag". Then ask yourself whether this particular concern is something over which you have control. If the answer is "NO", then write it down on a piece of paper, fold it up, and throw it in the bag. Throwing our worries in the bag is tantamount to giving them up to God. No sense attempting to play God, which, of course, just adds another set of impossible problems to the list. If it's out of our control, then it's up to God, its in God's hands.

4. There will be times when we will worry about some of the

items despite the fact that we've placed them in the bag. When (and notice I said 'when') we do this, we should take that particular item out of the bag until we're ready to put it back. In this way the bag also becomes a ritual of awareness that can help us spot those elusive control tendencies. The bag can be used for concerns within our control as well, but is especially useful for the others.

5. Medication may be helpful in opening a window of opportunity for practicing what we've learned when we just can't do it ourselves in spite of our knowledge and faith. This can be a useful temporary measure; so that we can slow down enough to practice the above outlined attitudes and behaviors. Of course, we need toconsult our physician in this regard. Medication here refers to medicine specifically designed to treat anxiety, depression, and sleeplessness.

Regardless of what we call this fear-nervousness, anxiety, or worry…it stems from a misunderstanding regarding the best strategy for dealing with discomfort. It is more useful to spend time *with* our emotional and spiritual discomfort, than to *avoid* it. We will begin to experience relief, as we are better able to manage, and perhaps even master our fears, anxieties and worries. We are bound to feel more "in control" and competent. Again, we encounter paradox and contradiction. For, it is only when we let go of control that we truly begin to experience control.

Summary

- The uncertainty of unknown outcomes provokes fear. The intensity levels of our fear vary from nervous tension to sheer terror.

- We often function in our daily lives as if we have complete control and are insulated from all misfortune. Complete control, however is an illusion.

- A pattern of social isolation creates more problems than it solves.

- Avoidance of fear and discomfort breeds more of the same. This common sense strategy is actually counter to our goal of increased security and control.

- Worry is a futile attempt to control the future.

- Compartmentalizing worry can help us limit its interference. Writing, the God Bag, and anti-anxiety medication are other useful fear management tools.

- Living in the present moment and having faith in long-term outcomes allows us to feel calmer and more secure.

- Letting go of control is the key to acquiring it.

This book is INTERACTIVE…

Fear can be paralyzing…What would it mean to you to have the ability to feel the fear, but do it anyway?

To get access to more resources visit…

http://michaelgusac.ibi3g.com/MYBK9

Part Three

The Plan

TURN DOWN THE VOLUME

The Central Attitude

STRESS MANAGEMENT INVOLVES our awareness of the whole person. As a consequence, attention must be paid to emotional, physical, spiritual, and mental health. There is an attitude that enables us to most effectively utilize the multitude of skills offered and the encyclopedic information available related to maintaining our optimum level of health as we limit our stress levels. This is an attitude that makes it likely that we will persist and succeed in our recovery.

The attitude, quite simply, is making self-nurturing (i.e., taking good care of ourselves) a high priority on our personal list of needs and wants. To consistently manage our stress level requires that we take the time and make the effort to maintain our tension levels in a healthy balance (be they physical, emotional, or spiritual). We will only do this if we believe that it is sufficiently important, if we believe that *we* are sufficiently important to justify the effort, to justify postponing certain items on our daily "to do" list in order to create the necessary time required for relaxation. Learning to relax, to "turn down the volume", is the central challenge of stress management.

Stress Defined and Described

What exactly is stress? Stress is experienced when we *perceive* ourselves to be threatened *and* do not feel *adequate* to handle the threat.

The physiological, stress response is familiar to us all: increased heart rate, increased breathing rate, increased muscle tension, surface cooling of our extremities, increased blood pressure, increased sweating, and tightness in the stomach and chest are some of the symptoms. Now the threat need not be physical (which is what this primitive stress response was originally designed to address); remember it can be any *perceived* threat. Certainly, if a bear is charging us we perceive a very real threat to our life. But imagine that you hear a noise in the dark of the night. The stress response triggers as your heart pounds. "Has someone broken in? Is it a burglar? Am I in danger?" you wonder. You discover that it's your dog trying to get into the garbage can in the kitchen. You breathe a sigh of relief as you think, "I'm not in danger after all!" It was the perception of a potential threat and your uncertainty about your ability to overcome the threat that triggered your pounding heart. And it was your realization that it was "only the dog" that calmed you down…the relaxation response…the perceived threat evaporated.

The fears and worries to which we referred in the previous chapter apply here as well. As we anticipate pain or an encounter with an unsympathetic health care provider, we react with varying degrees of nervous tension, finding these events more or less worrisome (translate *stressful*) depending on our perceptions. Or as we wonder whether the test results bode well or ill, the anticipation is stressful to varying degrees. We may become irritable. Emotional reactivity tends to be greater when we feel pressured and stressed.

Stress can also result from more objective impositions, such as too much noise or persistent pain levels (you may remember that I connected pain with stress in the introduction). There may be financial problems. Our injury/illness may affect our ability to be sexually intimate. We may be criticized at work or home if our productivity suffers as a consequence of our limitations Persistently high levels of stress contribute to a variety of medical problems. Heart conditions, hypertension, ulcers, and headaches are some of the obvious examples. Stress can compromise our immune system functioning as well. It is difficult to recuperate if constant stress and tension emotionally and/or physically exhaust us.

All stress is not necessarily bad. Hans Selye even coined a term for positive stress…"Eustress", as opposed to "Distress". An example might be getting married, or buying a car. Good stuff, but stressful nonetheless. Stress is unavoidable. Good or bad, positive or negative, it's part of our daily life. But what's relevant for us is the way it affects our health, given that our illness, pain, or injury is already quite challenging. How can we best address the effects of stress? Let's consider relaxation.

The Relaxation Response

It's time to "Turn down the volume", and to integrate relaxation into our daily routine. Hopefully we have learned that avoidance and pretending to ignore challenges and unwanted news (and stress can qualify as such), is not a viable approach. Relaxation can interrupt, if not reverse, the destructive aspects of stress related to constantly living with the challenges of our illness or injury. We don't have to be "miserable". The "relaxation response" researched by cardiologist Dr. Herbert Benson describes the reversal of the stress response symptoms. As we relax, our heart rate goes down, our muscles become more relaxed, and our extremities warm up…to name but a few examples. When we relax, our system actually releases morphine-like chemicals known as *endorphins* that can decrease our sensitivity to pain…or put another way, increase our pain tolerance.

This takes us back to that attitude I touched on at the beginning of this chapter. It's a question of priorities. In some ways this is an extension of the earlier chapter on pacing. We are exploring the approaches to our illness and injury that can help us be as active and productive as possible. And being as energetic and healthy as possible is what relaxation, stress management, and "turning down the volume" are all about. There is less emphasis here on productivity and more on health and nurturing ourselves. If "nurture" sounds too stuffy, then self care, or self-maintenance may be more appealing. But beyond the semantics, the point is that we have to consider our health as vitally important, and care for ourselves accordingly.

If we tend to do a better job of taking care of others than we do of ourselves, it can be difficult to shift the focus to our health. This is especially difficult for those of us who have been trained to be "caretakers". You Moms out there are a likely target for that type of training, although I don't want to exclude the guys from the caretaker role either. I've got a thought for all who struggle with this difficulty. We can just tell ourselves that this is for "them" (i.e. our loved ones). If we would feel too selfish and guilty to just "go fishing" for our own enjoyment and peace of mind, well then, do it for *them*. While we will certainly benefit (if we allow ourselves to do so), it is equally true that friends and family benefit when we are more cheerful and rested…less stressed.

We will probably have to put up with a little guilt in the interim. But if we "fake it" for a while and simply take the time to relax, we'll begin to experience some of the benefits of relaxation. Benefits such as: an increased energy level, serenity, a renewed sense of humor, a greater sense of control, fewer headaches, lower pain levels, and so on. The results help put the guilt in perspective. Now that we've committed ourselves to a program of stress management and relaxation, precisely what are we to do?

Approach and Intention

Well, I'm not convinced that the particular technique is as important as our approach, and our intentions relative to managing our stress levels. The approach I have in mind is well characterized by an ancient Chinese healing art known as Qi Gong (pronounced "Chi Gung"). It has been interpreted to me by Master Michael Lomax (apprenticed in Beijing, China, and now living near Jackson, Mississippi) that we can translate Qi Gong as "the study of energy that takes time and effort". Time and effort…that's the approach that works best.

Not magic, but rather persistence, patience and practice is the key. Consistent, regular practice virtually guarantees results; it's just a matter of time. Assuming we choose to integrate relaxation training into our daily routine, it's the disciplined routine that yields the most dependable results. Discipline, in its original Greek meaning, referred to *learning*, not to obligation and drudgery. As we "stick with it", we will get results. This is the "approach". What then is the "intention"?

The intention is self-healing, and self-nurturing. This means that it's not so much *what* we do as *why* we do it. Intention is a bit subtler than "why", but basically, anything that we're doing with the intention of taking care of ourselves counts as stress management and relaxation practice. The techniques are incredibly varied. There are no shortages of alternatives. Stress management and "wellness" has become a culture in its own right. But let's keep it simple.

I would suggest that if we're scrubbing the toilet, while telling ourselves that "this is for me"…perhaps a long avoided chore that is finally completed…then this is part of our practice, and our stress management program. Admittedly, I'm pushing this a bit to the extreme. I would hope that we could come up with something a bit more entertaining, but the nature of our *intention* is the point. At any rate, the method, the activity needn't be a formal meditation or relaxation technique. A walk in nature, a phone call to a friend, a soak in the tub, reading the Bible or a good book can all satisfy the goal...it depends on our reasons, on our intentions.

A Few Specific Suggestions

To conclude this section, I can't help but share a few personal favorites. Pick up a book on Qi Gong, and seek out an opportunity to have someone teach it to you. Take a Tai Chi class, and see what that is like. Walking is great for healing what ails us (there's a reason why they make us get up and walk the day after surgery). Consider Yoga, painting, reading, cycling, or coffee with a friend...anything you would find relaxing and enjoyable. And, if you do nothing else, take two minutes out of your day and practice breath awareness by learning to master the technique of diaphragmatic breathing.

The diaphragm is the muscle that forms the floor of our chest cavity and is designed to do 80% of our breathing. It is wired to our heart by our nervous system, and will slow down our heart rate as the breathing slows down. In diaphragmatic breathing, we limit the use of our shoulder and chest muscles. Our stomach expands like a balloon when we inhale and goes flat when we exhale (it's the reverse with chest breathing). Work toward slowing down the breathing pattern to 4 seconds per inhale and exhale. Breathe naturally, just slower. Put one hand on the chest and one on the abdomen to track progress. Just a few breaths should do it. Once we're good at it, even three complete breaths will make us lightheaded (too much oxygen). This won't hurt us, but two is quite sufficient. By all means keep your breath in your tummy after having taken the complete breaths; just breathe in a shallower, more natural rhythm (i.e. a bit faster).

I share this particular technique in some detail, because I get more positive reports from clients about this tool than all of the other ones I teach. Breath is incredibly powerful! It is also easily accessible, and readily available...whether we're walking from here to the water fountain, at a stoplight, or in the middle of an argument when the other person is talking (this one, of course, takes greater skill and concentration). Essentially…it's quick, and it works. We don't need 20 minutes of quiet time for this gem; 20 seconds is closer to what's actually required to get results.

I would recommend doing the breathing practice a minimum of five times per day. This only adds up to two minutes a day. Two minutes that will create a habit of breathing which will: (1) decrease your physical reactivity to stress (2) increases the oxygen concentration in your blood stream and (3) slow down your heart rate. And as part of your five times, do it a few times when you don't necessarily need to do it. This way your body will go beyond just getting back to normal to actually becoming relaxed.

So practice, and enjoy learning and relaxing. And remember, if you want to successfully "turn down the volume", you'll have made it a part of your daily routine. This goes beyond just putting out fires. This is to help blow out the match before the fire ever starts. Prevention is the larger goal.

Summary

- It is important to make relaxation a high priority.
- Stress is experienced when we perceive our coping skills as inadequate to the perceived threat.
- Persistently high levels of stress can lead to medical problems.
- Stress is unavoidable. It can be positive as well as negative. Positive stress is called Eustress. Negative stress is called Distress.
- The relaxation response can reduce our pain and reverse the immediate effects of the stress response.
- Consistent stress reduction practice yields the most dependable and beneficial results.
- Diaphragmatic breathing is an excellent technique for decreasing stress levels.
- Blow out the match, so you don't have to put out the fire.

This book is INTERACTIVE...

Are you struggling with tension, stress, and anxiety?

To get access to more resources that can deepen your ability to relax visit...

http://michaelgusac.odgi.net/MYBK10

THE INEVITABLE IS COMING! BETTER PLAN FOR IT

Balanced Optimism

I KNOW THE title of this section is a bit redundant. If it's inevitable, then of course it's coming. While that may appear to be an obvious connection, it's surprising how easy it is for us to pretend that we'll never have any bad days. Now there is clearly a certain utility in carrying on in spite of our illness or pain, in learning to live with it. But this is, as always, a question of balance. At least in the early stages of learning to manage a chronic condition, our natural tendency is to "hope for the best". And it is our belief that in so doing we are choosing optimism and acceptance. This is true to a point. However, as we progress and mature in our recovery and in our adjustment to living with a chronic condition, we'll "know we're there" when we come to the point of evolving both a relapse prevention plan, and a "flare" plan.

A "flare-up" refers to the physical aspects of our condition. For example, our energy level, our pain level, and the symptoms associated with our illness or injury. Relapse prevention applies more to attitudinal, spiritual, and emotional factors that can affect our ongoing recovery and adjustment. Let's begin with the "flare" plan.

A Flare Is…

I came across this term as a trainer for the Lupus Foundation while facilitating educational groups focused on learning to cope with Lupus (an immune system illness that affects the connective tissue in our body…including many organs). A "flare" is a day, a week, or a month when our symptoms flare up and become more intense and more of an interference in our daily routine. What we would normally be able to do, given the limits of our illness and pain, is even more restricted.

We may be unable to do household chores, the laundry, or cook meals. We may not be able to mow the yard, to stay up as late as normal in the evening, or to play a game with our children. We may not be able to follow through with that commitment we made to go out to eat that evening with friends. We may have to limit our obligations; we may not be able to go to work. It's even possible that we may be reduced to staying in bed all day.

Clearly we all have to deal with these considerations, but often we only deal with them when it happens, without any prior planning. We are caught by surprise, as are those around us. This doesn't just affect us. I have learned that developing a plan for these days is very helpful for all concerned. So, with that in mind then, what do we do?

Employment Considerations

If our injury/illness allows us to retain our employment, we educate our employer on the nature of our illness or injury. We let the boss know that we may occasionally have to limit our work activity, or even go home. We let him/her know that we may be calling in sick more often now. Very often we avoid this communication, because we're concerned that the employer is going to think we are making excuses to avoid work. We may be worried that we're going to lose our jobs if we say anything about our limitations. But if it's reasonably possible, the best course of action is to keep our employer informed. We may be pleasantly surprised to learn that they are actually appreciative of our candor, and tend to make allowances in order to accommodate us. If we take the trouble to educate them on how to be supportive and helpful, they are often more than willing to work with us.

This is, of course, not always true. It is important to be prudent in the context of what we know of the management's history of administering personnel policies. While we need to be aware that we can never give anyone enough information to help them *fully* understand our incapacity, we can nonetheless do much in this regard. It is less confusing for all involved (and this includes colleagues and co-workers) when they understand that, at times, there will be things that we cannot do, although we *will* be able to do them on our better days. If we're not pretending that were better off than we are, and thus over extending ourselves to a point of exhaustion, then it will be more understandable when we are limited on our bad days. Others will better be able to understand the impact of our illness or injury if on those bad days we are both responsive to its' dictates and straightforward with them regarding how we are limited.

Family and Friends

We can also discuss with family and friends what a bad day is like and what we are, and are not, able to do on those days. Then friends are less likely to be offended when we have to call them up to cancel a scheduled meeting. Then our family is more willing to pick up the slack on a day when we cannot do our chores. However, keep in mind that most of us tend to be resistant to change. And thus, in their denial, family members and friends may drag their feet emotionally by reluctantly carrying out a task that would normally be ours to complete. This does not necessarily mean that they do not want to be helpful. This reluctance is a natural adjustment to change and uncertainty.

But our family and friends can only adjust to our limitations if we have traveled that path ourselves. We need to remind ourselves of the lessons we are learning about pacing, and begin to communicate this knowledge to them. However, we can't communicate this information effectively if we are overly apologetic or defensive while talking with them. We need to set an example for them by communicating in a matter of fact, "for your information" manner.

We will need to talk with those affected about how to allocate the chores on a flare day. That may be a day when it's paper plates and pizza…no cooking, and no dishes to wash. Even if no one is asked to do the additional chores, they need to understand that certain things will not get done on those flare days. We needn't be morbid or fatalistic as we discuss these issues with others. This is simply "The way it is" for today. We don't have to like it, but it is valuable to plan ahead and be prepared. Then when we do have one of those days, making the necessary adjustments and accepting the reality of the need to make those adjustments, helps things go a good deal smoother for all concerned.

Relapse Is…

A different aspect of our planning is addressed with the concept of relapse prevention. To my way of thinking, we are experiencing relapse when we "lapse" into the attitudes and reactions that are contrary to the wellness principles we have affirmed throughout this book. When we become overly controlling, when we "Lose the Balance", when we are not taking good care of ourselves, we are relapsing. When we overextend ourselves to the point of exhaustion, when we are grouchy, and when we go to any lengths to avoid discomfort, we are experiencing a relapse. A relapse prevention plan is based on the assumption that those days are unavoidable. And, if unavoidable, then it is wise to prepare for the inevitable.

The Nature of Change

It is helpful to understand the nature of change in order to most effectively interrupt relapse episodes. Change is not an event that happens, but an ongoing process. *Progress* is the realistic goal, *not* perfection. I would venture a standard of measurement: If we can successfully follow the recommendations made in this book 80 to 85 percent of the time, then we deserve an A+. We should not expect ourselves to do these things perfectly or with flawless consistency. Such expectations will lead to frustration. We will falsely conclude that we have "failed", when imperfection is in fact simply part of the human condition. We may conclude that we have been mistaken about our prospects for a meaningful and productive life. These conclusions can catapult us into rage or depression, which will further intensify any relapse episode.

We need to understand that we are bound to have bad days, attitudinally, emotionally, and spiritually. We had bad days when we were healthy and we'll have them again. Preparing for this is best done when we have our wits about us rather than in a moment of crisis. Otherwise we will find ourselves confused and unable to effectively respond. So let's explore how to create a relapse prevention plan.

Warning Signs and the Plan

The first step would be to simply identify warning signs progressively from early, to middle, to late stages. We should begin with very subtle signs, and then proceed to the most obvious. An example of an early warning sign might be noticing that we seem to be grouchy and irritable that day. A middle stage relapse sign might be our frustration compelling us to overdo, which intensifies certain symptoms associated with our injury or illness. A late stage warning sign might be the reoccurrence of a debilitating depression that isolates and immobilizes us. These examples need not necessarily fit into the category to which I assigned them…it depends on what fits individually for each of us.

Having then clarified the warning signs, we can begin to decide which interventions are most helpful. If applicable we can base our choices on what has worked well for us in the past. We should also consider including new interventions that we have not previously employed or considered. Think about actions such as how we talk to ourselves, or how we choose to think, or what we choose to do or not do. We may decide to postpone decisions and actions, or to distract ourselves so that there is sufficient time for us to regain our equilibrium. One thing that can be useful (assuming that we are aware that we are relapsing) is to be generous with ourselves. It would be nice if we could maintain our health to perfection, but if we don't follow the guidelines in a particular instance, then at least we can learn from our mistakes, and be a bit more consistent in the future. We must be careful when we tell ourselves that we "shouldn't" be behaving in a particular manner. Insofar as it helps heighten our awareness that there's a problem requiring our attention (if not intervention), the word is useful. But with any "should" follows a value judgment that is usually negative and selfcritical. I am reminded of a phrase I heard at a symposium a few years ago that caught my attention: "Don't should on yourself, it will make you feel *shouldy*." Take responsibility for change, but don't take on unnecessary guilt. We do the best we can. We resolve to persist so that we can become more consistent in the attitudes and behaviors that we have come to understand will most contribute to our adjustment and recovery. If we do some realistic planning for our bad days, both spiritually and physically, what we discover is not that, because we are thinking about it, those days seem to happen more frequently, but that in doing the planning, we are better prepared and more at ease. The flare-ups and relapses that we do experience tend to be less intense and of shorter duration.

The List

I strongly encourage you to write your plan down, and have it in a place where it's easily accessed. You might even want to have something you can put in your purse or wallet. That way, if you begin to relapse, you'll be ready for action. Don't trust your memory in this regard, because if you hit a particularly rough spot, you're going to have a hard time thinking straight. But if you can see what you have written down in some of your best moments, you can simply do it, regardless of whether you think it's a bright idea at the time. Then, if nothing else, you're occupied, distracted, and engaged in a solution. This in itself can be quite beneficial. To have some direction and know what needs to be done can be a great help.

Once again, even if we don't do it at the time, to know what we need to do is the "beginning". Awareness is the beginning of change. The activity of writing this list can also help us heighten our awareness in specific ways that increase the likelihood that we will spot the warning signs when they occur. This stuff can creep up on us very quickly, if we're not careful. We don't need to look over our shoulders with a frightened sense of paranoia, but at the same time we can be too cocky, even on the good days. Sooner or later, there are going to be some rough spots. Life's going to throw us a curve, our symptoms are going to intensify, and we will fall back into familiar, but currently unproductive, patterns of thought or action. If we can spot the warning signs then, at least, we have the opportunity to prepare. If we're operating out of habit (which often happens), the value of a piece of paper to which we can refer every now and then in order to help us catch ourselves can be immeasurable.

So, in conclusion, the relapse prevention plan can help us crystallize and formalize our understanding as we integrate the lessons of this book. One other note: the plan can be flexible. We just need an initial blueprint from which to work. We can make revisions as time goes along, as we change, as circumstances indicate. We are well on our way to a productive adjustment to our illness or injury.

Summary

- Pretending we'll never have any bad days is an unbalanced optimism.
- A flare-up refers to a worsening of our physical symptoms.
- Educating our employer on the ups and downs of our condition can improve our working relationship with him/her.
- Straightforward communication with family and friends can help prepare all concerned for the bad days.
- Relapse is when we lapse into attitudes and reactions that do not support Wellness.
- Progress, not perfection is a realistic recovery goal.
- Soaking in guilt is self-indulgent. Admit your mistakes, but then take the opportunity to learn from them.
- A list of progressive relapse warning signs can help us choose the most appropriate intervention.

This book is INTERACTIVE…

You want to be able to deal with the realities of living with the persistent challenges of chronic pain and illness…

To access more resources…

http://michaelgusac.ibi3g.com/MYBK11

DON'T JUST SURVIVE... THRIVE!

Stress Management

I HAVE MENTIONED on numerous occasions in the text that the focus of this book is on attitude rather than the detailed "to do" specifics. We've discussed my conviction that if we have the right attitude then, in many ways, the details will take care of themselves. Of course, it helps to have an information base from which to draw. That's why I've provided you with a brief bibliography of additional reading resources at the end of the book. This is also why I'm going to go into some detail on various techniques that I teach my clients in order to enable them to more effectively manage their injury/illness. Additionally, my colleagues and friends encouraged me to outline some of these techniques. You can use the Table of Contents for quick reference once you develop your preferences. Given the vast range of available offerings, this may help you refine your search.

Breath Awareness

Technique 1: Diaphragmatic Breathing—Let me begin by simply reaffirming the value of diaphragmatic breathing and utilizing breath as a tool in managing stress. This was included in the chapter entitled *Turn Down the Volume*. Please refer to this chapter for a detailed treatment of this technique (P. 88). I have found that this procedure, above all others, stands the test of time. My clients will maintain it as part of their daily routine when all the other techniques may have been neglected.

Let me also suggest some other things that can be done with the breath, which can help you in your day-to-day efforts at coping with your injury/illness. Don't underestimate the usefulness and power of breath work. There is no better tool to re-establish balance in your nervous system. Give any of these techniques a two-week trial.

Technique 2: Breath Counting—I learned this initially as a meditation method associated with Zen Buddhism. It can be used as a tool to help you get to sleep, to help you relax in general, and also as a tool to help develop concentration. The technique involves following your breath on *both* the inhalation and the exhalation. As you're following the breath, count "One" on the inhalation and "Two" on the exhalation, and follow this through sequentially to the count of "Ten". When you get to "Ten", then begin your count over again. Do this repeatedly for about 10 minutes.

You may discover that you occasionally lose count. For example, as you count "four" and find yourself wondering whether you already counted "three". If this happens, you may either return to the beginning by starting over again at "One", or (and this is my recommendation) simply move on to the next number. One other indicator that you have lost count, is when you suddenly notice that you just counted "Seventy" because you didn't stop when you got to "Ten". Here, I *would* recommend that you return to the beginning and start with "One".

While our ability to take the count from one to ten repeatedly may be useful as an indication of our level of concentration, the counting is primarily a tool to enable us to follow the breath. You will get better at maintaining your count over time, but watching the breath is our initial purpose. If you're using this to help you manage sleep disturbance, losing count is, in fact, a *good* sign…a sign that you're falling asleep. However, when you are using breath counting to calm yourself or focus your mind, then at least approximating the count is valuable.

There are some ways of making this practice more challenging. In this way we are using the breath counting to deepen our relaxation practice, quiet the mind, and focus our concentration: (1) *Begin* your count on the *exhalation* rather than on the inhalation as you count to "Ten". This approach is a less natural and intuitive way of breathing, and thus takes a bit more concentration. You are still counting on *both* the in and out breath, but you reverse the order as in breaths are now the *even* rather than the *odd* counts. Example: *Inhale* (No count), *Exhale* ("One"), *Inhale* ("Two"), *Exhale* ("Three"), and so on. (2) More difficult than #1 above is the technique of counting only on the inhalation, and skipping the count on the exhalations. (3) And most difficult is the method of counting only on the exhalation, and skipping count on the inhalations. All the counts are 1-10.

Save these more challenging techniques for your practice as you progress over time, and begin with the breath counting in its simplest version for insomnia and learning to relax. It can also become a form of meditation to calm the mind. It can be done sitting, lying down, standing, or walking. In fact, one of my favorite forms of practice is to count my breath while I walk. The breath can be used to coordinate your pace (e.g. a left step on each inhalation…or every other inhalation). And keep your eyes open, of course, and pay attention while you're walking. It would take all the fun out of your practice if you fell and injured yourself in the midst of all this wonderful stress management stuff.

Technique 3: *Breath Imagery-Words and Phrases*…Use your creative abilities and imagine that as you breathe *in*, you are breathing in *relaxation*, and as you breathe *out* you are breathing out tension. So it's relaxation *in*, and tension *out*, in a nice, natural, easy breathing rhythm. You can use whatever words might create the associations that would be the most useful for you at any given time. For instance, you might prefer *comfort in*, and *discomfort out*…or *serenity in*, and *worry out*. Basically, the concept is…positives *in*, and negatives *out*. Make an effort to really feel the positive attribute coming in with the breath, and to really feel the unwanted attribute leaving with each exhalation. Use your imagination…it can be surprisingly powerful.

You might also find it valuable to integrate or coordinate a phrase with your breathing pattern. A phrase such as…"Let It Go", "Take It Easy", "Thy Will Be Done". Here we're combining the breath with positive self-talk, positive self-statements. For example: "Let it" (Inhale), "Go" (Exhale)…or "Take It" (Inhale), "Easy" (Exhale). You will find them to be more powerful and effective when used in this manner.

Technique 4: *Breath Imagery-Color*…You may also use your creative powers to enhance a soothing sense of relaxation and calm by imagining that you are inhaling a color of your choosing. Perhaps it's your favorite color…perhaps it's simply whatever color first comes to mind. Allow that color to fill you up as if you were a glass being filled with water. When you are colored inside from head to toe, imagine that the color is then soaking through to the surface until your skin is that color as well (imaginatively speaking of course). Notice the sensations associated with becoming the color…and the thoughts…and the emotional reactions.

Autogenics

This method uses self-suggestions or statements to evoke the relaxation response. You can use images to create various physical sensations, which can then benefit your system in various ways. One variation of this technique is to develop a sensation of warmth in your limbs. This is designed to improve circulation, as well as provide a general decrease in muscle tension levels. This is based on our understanding that mind and body are so intimately connected that if we think about warmth, we will actually become warmer physically.

The procedure: Begin by taking a few deep breaths. As you inhale, hold your breath for as long as is comfortable, and then fully exhale while gently tightening the abdomen to expel any remaining air. Repeat this once more. Then silently repeat to yourself the following: "My left arm is warm…My left arm is warm…My left arm is warm."[2] Then slowly repeat three times: "My right arm is warm…My right arm is warm…My right arm is warm." Then slowly repeat three times: "Both my arms are warm." Then repeat this series with your legs: three times with your left leg, and then with your right leg, and finally both legs. End by suggesting to yourself: "I am relaxed" as you let the relaxation deepen and the warmth spread.

Explore your own experience and discover what type of sensation is most relaxing for you. Perhaps you would want to imagine sensations of weightlessness. Or perhaps you would prefer sensations of heaviness. Both of these sensations tend to be associated with muscle relaxation. Sensations of coolness might be more appealing to you.[3] Be creative with the images you use. Have fun with this! Experiment to see what works for you.

Progressive Relaxation

There are two types of progressive relaxation. One type is termed *active*; the other is termed *passive*. Active progressive relaxation involves actually tensing the specific muscle for a few moments, and then physically releasing and relaxing the muscle. As we do so, the muscles can become progressively more relaxed. A common example

[2] As you do this, you may use an image that's useful in assisting you to remember and experience this particular sensation (e.g. the memory of hands placed over a campfire, a hot shower or bath, or the sun shining on you arm at the beach).
[3] Many of us have used coolness for headache relief, or relieving pain from sunburn.

would be arching your back after a long spell of sitting, in order to stretch and relax the back muscles.

Passive relaxation involves focusing your attention on a particular muscle, and then directing your intention (will, desire) toward decreasing any tension that is noticed.[4] You may want to consider reading the following sample aloud and recording it on a cassette tape. You could then play back the dialogue as if someone else was guiding you through the experience. The language usage is somewhat different from normal, but will help facilitate a relaxed state.

Begin by following your breath as you imagine that you're breathing *in* relaxation, and breathing *out* tension…Really *feel* the relaxation coming in with the breath, and the tension leaving as you exhale.[5] Do this again. Now just let your breathing take care of itself…and notice the muscles in your feet…in your toes…your arches…and let go of any tension that you notice. There's no need to *make* the muscles relax, just *allowing* them to relax…just *letting* them relax…a kind of *effortless* effort. And as your feet are relaxing, you can begin to notice the muscles in your calves…just letting go of any tension that's there…allowing your calf muscles to relax. And as your feet and calves begin to relax, you can notice the muscles in your thighs…letting go of any tension that you notice there, as your thigh muscles become relaxed…and you become *more* and *more* relaxed…feeling calmer…more serene. And you can notice the muscles in your stomach and chest…as your breathing *in* relaxation, and breathing *out* tension…letting go of any tension that's there…allowing those muscles to relax…becoming *more* and *more* relaxed… that's right! And you can notice the muscles in you fingers…allowing them to relax…comfortable and relaxed…as your fingers and arms

[4] I favor this style in my practice; particularly for clients who are experiencing problems due to muscle tension and spasms related to their injury or illness. Often the muscles are already behaving in an unhealthy manner by holding on to tension once they are activated.

[5] In this dialogue (…) means pause for 1-2 seconds…whatever feels like a gentle relaxed pace. Don't rush!

become *completely* relaxed. And you can notice the muscles in your neck and shoulders…and any tension you notice there…just letting go of that tension…*effortlessly* and *automatically*. And as your neck and shoulders relax, you can notice the muscles in your scalp…allowing those muscles to relax. Perhaps you notice a slight tingling sensation as those muscles relax…and you become *more* and *more* relaxed. That's right. And as your scalp muscles relax, you can notice the muscles in your face…around your eyes and mouth…just letting go of any tension you notice there…so that as your face becomes smooth and relaxed, you can also notice the muscles in your jaw. And as your jaw muscles relax, and your jaw drops slightly, you can become *completely* relaxed. And you can just idly wonder how that feeling of relaxation and peace can spread and deepen…becoming *more* and *more* relaxed. Just taking a few minutes now to be silent…and feeling calm and relaxed.

And then whenever you're ready…and you'll know when that is…just beginning to reorient yourself to your surroundings as you open your eyes (if they were, in fact closed)…so that as you notice what you see you can become more alert. And as you notice what you see, and any sounds you hear you can feel more refreshed. And as you notice what you see, hear, and sense…perhaps the temperature on the surface of you skin…you can feel more energized as well. Alert…Refreshed…and Energized…resolved to play with this practice whenever you feel the need…as often as you like.

Insomnia

Sleep disturbance is a common problem when chronic pain and illness are involved. It can be difficult to fall asleep, and it can be difficult to remain asleep. If our pain awakens us, it is often difficult to return to sleep. We already mentioned in the section on breathing practice that breath counting could be used as a technique for falling asleep when we're having difficulty doing so. You might consider it advanced sheep counting. Let me mention a couple of other techniques that I've found useful over the years.

Technique 1: Turn Down The Volume...If you're having trouble getting to sleep, and the interference happens to be a lot of inner mind chatter, this technique may be useful. Imagine a dial that is marked from 1-10, similar to what you would find on a radio dial. As the chatter is distracting, and interfering with your sleep pattern, you can imagine that the inner dialogue is *loud* and *fast* paced...and thus the volume level on the dial is at "10". The strategy is to turn down the dial incrementally, one number (one level) at a time. As you do this, wait until you actually experience the chatter becoming *a little bit* quieter and slower in pace. As this happens, and only *when* this happens, turn the volume down another notch on your imaginary dial...see the dial moving only *after* you've experienced the change. Then progressively turn down the volume so that at perhaps 4 or 5, the chatter is so much less of interference that you can fall asleep. Perhaps you fall asleep in the midst of the exercise. Wouldn't that be nice?

It's important that you actually experience each change before you see the dial moving in your mind's eye. If you find that your imaginary dial is at a 5, but the chatter is at 10, then you should never have gone past 9...you didn't really wait for the actual experience of quieting and slowing.

Regardless of how skilled you become with this technique, there will be nights when you just can't quiet your mind. Now, it can also happen that the volume can go back up to a 10 after having been at a 5, but that is different from never having noticed a change at all. If this happens, then cycle through the process again, and see if you can quiet your mind once more.

Technique 2: Erasing The Blackboard...Imagine a blackboard, or a whiteboard, or a greenboard...but whatever the color, imagine that the mental chatter that is cycling through your mind is being projected up onto the board. See the text (thoughts) scrolling down from top to bottom until the entire board is full. Then you imaginatively erase that board. As you do that, the board will begin to fill again with all the chatter that's streaming through. Just let it show up on the board, and as it does, calmly erase it away. This clears the board for yet another board full of script to appear. It's almost as if you were flipping through single frames in a motion picture.

If this procedure works, the speed with which the words appear on the board becomes slower and slower. Then you notice there is a point at which the board is no longer filling up, that whatever shows up on the screen, once erased, does not refill. The board is blank, your mind is quiet, and you're prepared for some restful sleep. It's not absolutely necessary that the board is blank for you to be able to sleep. In fact, you easily may fall asleep even as the appearance of words begins to slow.

Technique 3: Erase Yourself... This is similar to progressive relaxation as you start with your feet and progress up your body to your head. Imagine that you are erasing (making invisible...or eliminating) your body one section at a time. You may notice a feeling of relaxation or numbing either prior to, or immediately following the erasure. The physical sensations and the image coincide, and thus complement and deepen the experience. By the time you get close to the neck and shoulder region...you're probably already asleep.

Technique 4: Journaling... This is a good way of dealing with worry and anxiety which is what mind chatter often happens to be. As you write down your thoughts, it tends to slow them down. The thoughts are objectified so they can be examined dispassionately. Perhaps new insights occur. If you still can't sleep, you can at least enjoy the satisfaction of spending that time constructively. When you are feeling quite fatigued, then return to bed, hopefully without the repetitive, restless thoughts that have been keeping you awake.

Bubble Up

In the interest of stress management, here's a method of coping with tension, anxiety, or fear... *The Technique*: Begin by relaxing as you follow the breath, imagining that you are breathing in relaxation and breathing out tension...breathing in calm confidence, and breathing out fear and worry. Allow your mind to drift as you remember an experience...a place (perhaps in nature) where you felt safe and secure. If nothing seems to come to mind, then invent a place that appeals to you and could provide that sense of protection. Allow this place to become as vivid and real as possible.

Now imagine a bubble surrounding you in a color that appeals to you...whatever first comes to mind. If a bubble feels too fragile to provide protection, then imagine a force field. Project this protection out at about arm length (3-6 feet), and have it completely envelop you all around...above, below, front, back, right, and left. You can then imbue this barrier with whatever functions are most useful for you. It can provide protection in the sense of *repelling* threats, stresses, and attacks. It can protect you by *reflecting* negative influences like critical insults. It can also be thought to *insulate* you inside a field of protection. Thus your bubble can provide the simultaneous functions of both insulation and repulsion/reflection. Allow the feelings of security and confidence to completely penetrate you. And then, whenever you need to reclaim this feeling, this confident sense of serenity and security, imagine your bubble. In an *instant*, protection and safety are yours. Strange perhaps, but effective.

The Word

Have you ever had the experience of hearing a song that reminded you of a particular moment in your life...perhaps a moment of romance, of success, or exhilaration? If music was not the stimulus, then some other environmental event that triggered a particular memory? Well, "The Word" operates according to the mechanism that accidentally connects events in our life with environmental stimuli. This type of memory is virtually (and some believe *actually*) imprinted at a *cellular* level. It is impressed on us, imbedded in us in a way that allows the environmental trigger to consistently elicit the memory every time it is present. This is true of traumatic memories (e.g. a life threatening injury or being robbed at gunpoint), as well as of the more positive moments in our lives.

This procedure *deliberately* and purposefully utilizes this phenomenon of memory imprinting to create a key to accessing positive experiences in our lives that can function as resources for us in much the same way that we would call a friend for advice, consolation or reassurance. We can instantaneously access these resources through recalling a word that can trigger these thoughts and feelings that are be useful to us.

Here then is *The Procedure*:[6] Begin by focusing on your breath, and imagine that you are breathing in relaxation, and breathing out tension…getting into a nice, easy rhythm…effortless…automatic…relaxing. Just doing that for a few moments now…and then just putting your breathing on autopilot…just let it take care of itself. And then, without really looking for it…just whatever comes to mind…allowing a memory to occur…of a time…an experience that can be useful to you as a resource…a solution for a problem or situation that is currently of concern to you (for example, if you're anxious, a memory of a time when you felt confident and able to handle any challenge).

As you become more and more relaxed…recalling that moment…just taking all the time you need…allow yourself to be *in* this memory. You're not watching yourself as if you were on stage…you're actually *in* it. And because you're *in* this memory…you can look all around…to the front, the sides, above, below…noticing

---

[6] Once again, as with the progressive relaxation technique, you may want to record a tape that could help you most effectively relax into this as you listen to it.

colors, shapes, size…the play of light and shadow…in as much detail as possible as you casually survey all around. And moving from one item to another, just seeing what you can see. And as you see what you can see…you can also notice what you *hear*…sounds from any direction…and whether the sounds are high or low…loud or soft…fast or slow paced…in as much detail as possible without too much time spent on any particular item. And the silence between the sounds…and how loud or soft the silence is. And you can notice any *odors* in this experience as you're *in* it…fresh, clean…whatever you notice, coming from any direction. And you can notice any *tastes*, as you're *in* this experience…sweet, sour…salty…whether your mouth is wet or dry. And then noticing the *sensations* you feel, as you're *in* this experience…warm, cool…wet, dry…rough, smooth…as you come in contact with your surroundings, and your surroundings come in contact with you…the feel of your clothes perhaps…as you're *in* this experience.

And as all the different parts of this experience come together, also noticing the *emotions* and feelings that are associated with this experience…and the *thoughts…attitudes…perspectives*…that come with the feelings and sensations…sounds and sights. And as all of this comes together now, and becomes most *vivid*…just allowing a *word* to occur that can connect with and represent this experience…just noticing whatever first comes to mind…taking all the time you need…allowing sufficient time for a good connection to be established between the word and the experience. Then gradually open your eyes, feeling alert, refreshed and energized as you reorient yourself to the room your present surroundings.

Now that you've completed this procedure, you can verify its effectiveness by recalling "The Word" later that day in order to see what effect you notice. Is there a noticeable shift in your mood, your attitude, and the physical sensations of your body? If not, I would suggest spending a few minutes before you go to bed each night for a week or so and notice some additional details that will make the experience more vivid, more real.

It's important to note that the Word is not intended to help you remember the experience, and then the thoughts and feelings. No… The Word that has occurred to you is a direct, immediate, instantaneous link to that moment when the experience peaked. As quickly as snapping your fingers…there it is.

This need not necessarily be used in a moment of tension or conflict. If you're feeling tired, you might recall the Word in order to provide an energy boost. If you're sad or depressed, you might use it to elevate your mood. You could even use it in conjunction with most any technique in this section, since it is so quickly accessible, once mastered. The possibilities are endless.

Pain

If these techniques work for you, they will work because of the body/mind connection to which we have referred throughout this book. The Mind/brain and body are connected in a way such that each affects the other. As you begin each of the exercises, it is as if your pain is talking to you as it represents itself as an image or impression. Then as you attempt to alter the image or impression using your imagination, it's as if you are talking back to your pain or discomfort, and it is willing to listen. Don't bother agonizing over whether this is "all in my head"…if it works, use it.

You may benefit by altering your vocabulary a bit, and labeling your pain as *discomfort*. It's amazing how much difference a single word can sometimes make! This simple word choice can actually encourage a different interpretation of our pain sensations. Pain is less your "enemy" when thought of as "discomfort". If you are willing to listen to your pain, it is more likely to listen to you. I know this is anthropomorphizing the pain, but, if chronic, it is your *companion* whether you like it or not. I know these techniques can reduce your pain levels...I've seen and experienced it personally on countless occasions. It may take practice, and some techniques will work better for you than others, but I assure you it's well worth the effort.

Technique 1: Untying The Knot...We deal with muscular discomfort of many varieties. There are, for example, spasms, areas of sensitivity (sometimes called "trigger points" if they meet certain criteria), and areas of inflammation. Some muscle pain can be described as feeling like a tightly closed fist, or a knot. Use the image of the knot as a way of releasing tension and thus possibly effecting some reduction in the intensity of your pain.

Begin by taking a deep breath. Hold it as long as is comfortable, and then fully expel the air by tightening your abdomen as you come to the end of the exhalation. Take one more deep breath in this way. Send your attention to the area of discomfort, and visualize the muscle tightness in the painful region as a knot. See it in your mind's eye. Notice the type of material of which the knot is made...is it rope?...is it string?...is it nylon?...is it hemp? Is it smooth or rough? Notice the knot's color. Notice the knot's outline at the periphery. Notice how the strands in the knot weave in and out of each other.

Then use your imagination to begin to untie the knot. Develop a strategy for doing this, as you notice how the knot is tied and you decide which part of the knot you will first begin to untie. How much pressure will you need to apply? How tightly is the knot tied? As you find the best place to begin, notice what sort of resistance you encounter as the strands start to unravel? Notice any changes in shape as you see how the knot loosens and perhaps one strand separates from another. Really immerse yourself in the details. And as the knot begins to untie, be aware of how the physical sensations are beginning to change as well. Continue to untie the knot, doing this as deliberately as necessary and taking as much time as is necessary.

As the knot is finally untied, check in with the painful area, and see what you notice. Has the intensity of your pain decreased? If not, has "the edge" been taken off the intensity level? Or do you notice any change in your range of motion, your ability to move freely. Are you a bit more relaxed? Are you less upset about being uncomfortable? Anything counts! Everything is significant!

If you're unable to untie the knot during this visualization, you're free to use any tool at your imagination's disposal that would help. Perhaps you might use some pliers; perhaps you imagine cutting some strands with a knife…whatever has an effect if simply visualizing the change is not sufficient. Be creative! Play with this! Each episode of practice may be different…or it may be the same.

Technique 2: Spread The Pain…Locate the area of discomfort and notice the outline of this area as you draw an imaginary line around the periphery. Begin to allow this area to spread throughout your body. You can really begin to *feel* it diffusing. Use whatever method is useful in effecting this change. Perhaps you pretend you are pulling taffy, or spreading cake icing. Perhaps the diffusion resembles the way mercury splatters when a thermometer is broken.

As you conclude this exercise, there is no longer a pinpoint area of discomfort. If your pain level was a "5" in your knee, it may now be a "3" throughout your body. In some ways this may seem contrary to common sense or natural instinct. After all, you may say, "Why would I want to hurt everywhere?" "One location is bad enough!" But, if the intensity of the discomfort diminishes, it will be easier to go through your day, because your pain will be less distracting.

Technique 3: Pain Dissociation…In this procedure, you begin with an image of the pain, and then separate yourself from the image…or perhaps more accurately separate the image from you. To begin then: Take a couple of deep breaths as you hold the inhale as long as it's comfortable, and then slowly exhale until all the air is expelled by finally drawing in your abdomen to rid yourself of any remaining breath. Locate the area of discomfort. Notice the outer perimeter of the area. What is its *shape*?…Is it a square? Is it a rectangle? Is it a circle?…or some irregular shape? Is it three-dimensional...a ball or a cube? Now notice what *color* seems to be associated with this shape. Notice the *temperature* that's associated with this shape...is it warm...or cool? Notice whether there's any sensation of *weight* associated with this area...is it heavy...or light? Notice whether this image fits directly on the pain...is it larger than life...or smaller? Really see and feel all the details of this image. Let your pain talk to you.

Now that you are fully aware of the image, with an attitude of idle curiosity, wonder how this image could begin to move. The movement might be rapid, and it might be gradual...it might be smooth and it might be jerky. Just notice how you can move the pain with your imagination until it's about arm length "out there"... above, below, to the front or back...or the side. Once it's out there, let it grow until it's touching the ceiling and floor. Then shrink the image until it's the size of a quarter...out there. Then let it grow once more...this time just drifting off into the distance...toward the sun, the moon, the stars...as far as it wants to go...and perhaps it just goes "poof" into the distance...it just vanishes.

If you are unable to change the location, then play with the image wherever it happens to be. Pain, when severe, often tends to appear as hot, large, heavy, clear and distinct, and as the color red or black. If this describes your experience, then in order to lower your pain intensity levels, imagine the temperature changing...perhaps cooling off...and the color becoming less intense...a pastel perhaps. You may want to imagine the area as lighter...and smaller...and less distinct. Notice the sensations, and if they're intensifying rather than decreasing, then move these various aspects of the image/impression in the other direction. There are no rules for what your pain *should* be, or how it *should* represent itself.

If your imagination does not seem sufficient to effect a change, then use an imaginary tool. For example, use an imaginary paintbrush to mix in a different color...tie a helium balloon to it in order to make the pain image/impression lighter…or float it in water…or cool it off with some ice that draws the heat out as it melts.

Notice the aspects of the image and the nature of your pain experience as you conclude this technique. If the pain is not sufficiently diminished, then return to it fifteen or thirty minutes later and do it again. What changes do you then notice? If you have more than one area of discomfort, you could work with a different area of discomfort or work on several areas at the same time…whatever is useful. Be creative and playful, and see what you recognize. We may not be inclined to "play" with pain; but that sort of detached attitude can be as helpful as the practice itself. We'll be more flexible, creative, and effective. Our intervention choices will be more accurate and fitting. I know that at times *severe* pain may not allow such an attitude… just keeps this in mind. *Technique 4: Color Yourself*…Here we play exclusively with color. The difference between this technique and the one in the breath section is that we will focus on starting to do the coloring from the outside in, as opposed to the inside-out approach. This will make more sense in a

moment. This one can be fairly entertaining.

Begin by imagining that you are breathing in relaxation, and breathing out tension…breathing in *comfort* and breathing out *discomfort*. Just get into a nice, easy, natural rhythm…effortlessly and automatically relaxing. As you are relaxing pick your favorite color…or just see what color first comes to mind. Then pretend that you're dumping a five-gallon can of paint of that color on your head. Notice the sensations as gravity does its work and the paint begins to cover you from head to toe. It may stream down one side faster than another…just notice how it spreads, and how that feels. Just allow the paint to spread at its own pace. When you are finally covered, then allow the color to begin to soak in, both from the front and the back…and the top-bottom-sides until the color has met somewhere in the center of your body, and you become that color, both inside and out. Notice how you now feel…sensations…emotions…

thoughts. Notice the nature of your pain experience at this point. Is it somewhat less? Is it significantly less? Is it gone? Are you smiling? Are you relaxed? What do you notice?

If you prefer...or as an alternate procedure for coloring yourself...you could imagine that you are shining a spotlight on the area of discomfort...and then allowing the spotlight to turn into a flood light as the light covers your entire body. You turn around...or there are lights placed in different locations...so that you are fully covered by the color. As you are finally colored outside and inside, you can notice the effect. You can feel relaxed, reassured, serene, and in less pain...just see what shows up.

Technique 5: Expanded Focus...This procedure can be used with emotional, as well as physical pain. In order to work with emotional upset, locate a physical sensation that seems to correspond to a feeling..."butterflies" in your stomach, for instance, might be associated with nervousness. A weight on your shoulders could connect with feeling depressed. Anger might be associated with a flushed warming in your face. You get the idea.

Expanded Focus...(a) *Space*: For this practice, the initial dialogue is designed for a room in a house: Begin then by closing your eyes, and relaxing as you follow your breath and imagine that you are breathing in comfort and breathing out discomfort. That's right. Just get into a nice, natural, easy rhythm. And as you do so, locate an area of discomfort that you want to work with. Now imagine the *space* between that spot, and the front of your body. It may only be a paper-thin layer, but pretend there is some space between that spot and the outer surface of the skin. Then imagine the space between that spot and the *left* side of your body. When you've done that, imagine the space between that spot and the *back* of your body...and when you've done that...then imagine the space between that spot and the *right* side of your body...and then the *top* of your body... and then imagine the space between that spot and the *bottom* of your body. Now fill in any blanks so that you have a layer of space completely surrounding the area that used to be so uncomfortable.

Keep this layer in mind as you build a second layer of space around this uncomfortable spot. You have a layer of space surrounding the spot inside your body, and you are now going to imagine another layer of space surrounding your body. Imagine then a layer of space between your body and the *front* of the room. When you have done this, imagine a layer of space between the *left* side of the room and your body…and then a layer behind you…and to your *right*…and a layer between you and the *floor*…and a layer of space between the *ceiling* and you. Then fill in any gaps as you imagine a layer of space completely surrounding your body in the room. Now you have imagined a layer of space surrounding the area of discomfort inside your body, and then added a second layer surrounding your body in the room. Keep both of the layers of space in mind as you add one final layer.

Imagine a layer of space on the other side of the *front* of the room…heading out in that direction as far as it wants to go…off into the distance toward the horizon. Then, I wonder if you can imagine the space beyond the *wall* on the *left* side of the room, as far as it wants to go…off into the distance. And can you imagine the space beyond the *back* wall…as far as it can extend…and the *left* wall…and the *floor* heading toward the earth's core as far as it wants to go. And finally imagining the space *beyond the ceiling* as far as it wants to go toward the sun, the moon, and the stars. And then fill in the gaps so that there is a layer of space completely surrounding the room.

Now you have *three* layers of space surrounding the pain…a layer inside your body…a layer outside your body in the room…and a layer of space completely surrounding the room. Let your attention move from layer one…to layer two…to the space in the world beyond…and drift…as far as your attention wants to go. You may want to turn around and look at that small, insulated, insignificant spot so far away…or your attention may remain directed outward—the universe—beyond…just zooooming away. Now gradually open your eyes becoming alert, feeling refreshed and energized. Check in on your pain and see what you notice. And if it's emotional pain… how upset are you now?

Expanded Focus…Sound: We have worked opening our focus using *space* as the modality with which to work. *Sound* could be another modality to play with…although less focused on the pain location; it is a good way to expand our focus of attention. Briefly: Here we simply begin to notice the sounds in our surroundings. And as we attend to the sounds, we begin to focus on the hearing itself as the sounds begin to lose their labels…we are simply acquiring the experience of hearing as the sounds flow by like the drops of water that compose a mountain stream…one after another…sound after sound…and the silence between the sounds…and how loud or soft, high or low pitched the sounds can be…and how loud or quiet the silence can be. This is the basic opening of focus that can occur with sound…and silence.

Expanded Focus…Time: Time is one other mode in which we can play with opening our focus. For instance: How upset will you be about any particular conflict, any particular pain or upset five years from now? Will you even remember what was so upsetting ten years from now?[7] And how much were you hurting at this time yesterday? How much were you hurting a week ago at this precise moment in the day…or a year ago…seven years ago?[8] It can all be a matter of perspective. The larger temporal perspective can help us keep the present moment in perspective. This can be confusing… but enjoyable as well…it can keep us flexible…it can put our pain in the proper perspective. Albert Einstein liked to play with alternative <u>ways of conceiving</u> time…we're certainly in good company!

[7] Here, it's as if we're in the future (ten years from now), looking back at the past (today)…the present (now, this precise moment) becomes the past.
[8] Now it's as if we're in the past (seven years ago) looking toward the future (today)…the present moment now is transformed into the future.

Once you get a feel for opening your focus, you can invoke it almost instantaneously…much like "the Word" practice outlined earlier. When you are thoroughly familiar with it, you can get that zoom-out feeling with space, with sound, and with time (I'll let you discover how to open up other modes of perception…smell, size, touch, sight, etc.). I like to play with this when I go for walks… walking into the future or the past…zooming out to the far reaches of the universe, and so on. This brings me to the last tool I'm going to put in your tool kit…walking.

Walking

We've touched on walking in connection with several techniques already. It is one of my favorite activities because it's so universally beneficial. We've mentioned it in relation to breathing, in relation to the "open focus" practice, and as part of the prescription for remedying depression. It's prescribed immediately after many surgical procedures for a reason…it facilitates healing. It is gentle, and helps us maintain our range of motion. It regulates sleep and appetite… moving us in the direction of balance when we've had too much or too little. Walking is also useful for stress reduction.

Did you know that our spinal, skeletal, and muscular structures are actually designed for walking…not lying down, running, or sitting? Humankind has walked across continents over the generations of its history. Let me suggest some different ways of conducting your walks so that they remain interesting, thus increasing the likelihood that you will pursue walking with some regularity in a way that goes beyond exercise per se'. I'd very much like it if you got into a *habit* of walking.

Technique 1: *Noticing Differences*…When you go for a walk look for differences in your surroundings. Watch for a bird that wasn't there the day before. Watch for a piece of paper on the trail. Notice that tree that you've never *really* noticed before. We've all had those experiences where we saw something that had always been part of our surroundings, but had never quite *caught* our attention. This is good practice for developing your powers of observation and concentration. This is helpful in challenging the depressive habit of thinking that only notices what never seems to change. This also keeps your walks interesting. This is especially useful if you walk the same route daily.

Technique 2: Breath Awareness...Walking can become a form of meditation that quiets the mind, and soothes the spirit. Follow the breath as you walk. Notice how it fits with your pace. You can integrate the breath counting practice, or just use it to develop a quiet awareness. Notice how the breath can originate from your abdomen as you practice breathing diaphragmatically...this is your center...and you can feel *centered*.

Technique 3: Problem Solving...Many of us have had the experience of doing our best thinking when we "went out to get some fresh air". Use your walking time to sort through some problem or concern. This can become a constructive conclusion to an episode of worrying. You don't necessarily have to focus directly on a problem. Just leave your concern in the back of your mind as you walk...this is how we do some of our most creative thinking, when we have those "Ah Ha" experiences where the solution occurs when "we're not even thinking about it."

Technique 4: Body Awareness...While you are walking, take the opportunity to watch your body. Notice the mechanics of your movement. How do your arms swing from your shoulders? How do your legs swing out from your hips? Can you feel the movement in the joints? Notice how the muscles tense and relax. What areas of your body are more or less relaxed? How do you rock onto the balls of your feet from your heels? Can you keep your shoulders relaxed while you walk...even for long distances? What is your pace...How long does it take you to travel a certain distance? How does the walk affect your pain levels? Do you notice any change in your range of motion? And so on...

I would encourage you to walk daily...if only for five minutes.

Consistent daily walks will provide you more benefit than once or twice a week. If illness and/or pain levels allow, do more than just saunter when you walk. I'd recommend a moderate pace of 3mph. Walk aerobically if you like (which will be about 4mph). Pick a regular time, and then stick with it.

Conclusion

These various techniques place a good deal of emphasis on the use of your imagination, and on the use of visualization. It is my intention to provide a group of tools that have a broad range of applicability, and also provide a collection that draws on a variety of sources. As you explore these procedures, I encourage your doing so with an attitude of idle curiosity…or, if you prefer, an attitude of scientific experimentation. Have an open mind, and use them more than once in order to give yourself an adequate opportunity to discover their value to you. It is helpful to supplement the attitudes you are learning with the skills that can best actualize them.

Pain Management

Chronic illness/injury and pain are closely…often inextricably associated. Whether we focus directly on pain, or indirectly on relaxation and reducing stress…we are learning to take the edge off of our level of discomfort. We've also advocated attitudes that help us deal with pain in many of its forms (spiritual as well as physical). Now let us briefly touch on of the details of the physical mechanism of pain, and some of the devices and treatments available for pain relief. While attitude is the primary focus of our treatment, a foundation in the *detailed, technical stuff* can also be helpful. And while we are more focused on detail here, I only intend to draw outlines of *some* of the available pain treatments and devices.

Chronic vs. Acute Pain

We have discussed the fact that *chronic* conditions are distinguished from *acute* conditions according to the length of time one has had the problem. Chronic pain lasts for longer than three months. For most of us, an acute episode lasts only days…occasionally weeks, and rarely longer than a month. Surgery may be the occasional exception, but that also is often resolved within the month.

There are different physical pathways through which the brain interprets pain. One formulation of this observation has been called the "Gate Control" theory of pain. This theory utilizes our understanding that different types of nerves carry different types of pain impulses at varying speeds to the brain. There are two main pathways…one where impulses travel rapidly, and another along which the pain signals travel more slowly. This being true, the "Gate Control" theory explains how it happens that when you stub your toe, rubbing it seems to help reduce, even eliminate, the pain…at least while you're rubbing it. This happens because our rubbing stimulates neural pathways that move sensation impulses to the brain more quickly than the impulses arising from the injured area itself. The fast rubbing impulse gets to the brain before the slower stubbing impulse, and thus overrides the pain of the injury. It's as if a *gate* was closed, and the pain of the injury was shut off.

TENS Unit

There is a device called a TENS unit that utilizes the realities of the "Gate Control" theory. It electrically stimulates the brain as a *counterirritant*, so that while in use, while the unit is on and pushing an electrical impulse (powered by a 9-volt radio battery) the brain detects the artificially induced signal rather than the pain signal. While this is no cure, the TENS unit can provide welcomed temporary relief from the relentless pursuit of chronic pain. The electrical contacts are embedded in adhesive patches, which are placed locally on the painful area, and the current travels up the spinal column to the brain.

Some types of TENS[9] units have particularly high levels of current which are believed to stimulate one of the body's natural healing mechanisms. This is the mechanism we discussed in the chapter on depression where we reviewed the fact that the body can naturally produce morphine-like substances known as *endorphins*, which can decrease our sensitivity to pain. Here we are literally adding insult to injury in order to increase endorphin release. Parenthetically, let me add that claims are not typically made for the healing properties of these TENS units, rather they are promoted as simply providing temporary pain management. There are also devices that are designed to energize some of the same healing mechanisms with a gentler approach.

Gentle Stimulation Alternatives

Device 1: *Micro current Stimulation*…This particular type of electrical stimulation device is designed to match the electrical current that naturally flows through our nervous system. It is called micro current because the *frequency* (cycles per second…speed of signal transmission) is much slower than the traditional TENS units, and the *intensity* (amount of current push) is much less than that of most TENS units. The micro current frequencies are also thought to match brainwave frequencies that are associated with natural states of relaxation. These waves are in the range of approximately 8-12 Hertz (abbreviation Hz=cycles/second) and are called Alpha waves. As a result, there is often an experience of relaxation associated with this type of treatment when we place contacts on the skin surface.

9 TENS stands for Transcutaneous Electrical Neural Stimulation. Transcutaneous means "on the skin surface" and neural refers to nerves. the devices use adhesive patches to conduct the current.

Unlike traditional TENS units, the contacts are placed to go *through* the area of discomfort. Placing contacts on the back and abdomen, vs. exclusively on the back region, for example, would treat low back pain. It's as if the body was transparent, and we're running current through the pain. While these units are classified as TENS units because the stimulation is directed from the skin surface, the theory underlying their use is quite different. We are not using the Gate Theory and trying to "cover up" the pain. As this micro current goes through the pain it's as if we were using electrical current to unclog the electrical or energy pathways…to remove obstructions to the natural flow of current, thus allowing our physical system to return to a normal, healthy, pain-free equilibrium.

Device 2&3: *Ultrasound and Infratonic Therapy*…Here is another device that is based on the principle of actualizing the body's natural rhythms of current flow (energy/ electrical micro current) and circulation. The treatment is known as *infratonic* sound massage therapy. It again approximates the 8-12 cycles/second frequency. This time, however, it's the Alpha range of *sound* waves rather than waves of *electrical* current. These low frequency sound waves are known as *infrasonic* as distinguished from *ultrasonic* waves, which are the high frequency sound waves that generate a warming massage sensation. Both of these waveforms are beyond the human ear's ability to hear. Both can be beneficial. Experience is the judge.

The infrasonic massage is more gentle that ultrasonic with no risk of burning the skin surface. Neither does this type of treatment require the skin preparation that ultrasonic therapy requires. In fact, the treatment is often done 3-6 inches off the body's surface. This treatment is, for example, used in treating broken bone pain through the plaster cast. You can keep your clothes on, and place it either *on* or *away* from the body's surface. This is especially useful when you have a painful area that is sensitive to touch. This is a one of the more convenient forms of pain treatment.

If the therapy is helpful, it can improve circulation and nerve conduction. It can also reduce swelling and inflammation. It is thought to improve the functioning of the lymph system as well.10 [10]And, like micro current stimulation, the treatment is often reported to have a physically and emotionally relaxing effect on the individual.

Acupuncture

The "gentle" devices mentioned above are based on the same principal that the Chinese art/science of acupuncture is based. There are thought to be energy pathways which, when stimulated at certain points, can then remove obstructions to the natural flow of energy/current. They are in an intricate network/system, which does not necessarily correspond with nerve pathways. These energy pathways or channels are called "meridians". Very small gauge needles are used to activate these gateways and energy channels. As with the micro current and infrasonic treatments, if we reduce interference, the system's natural tendency toward health and balance will be actualized.

Acupressure

This treatment is also directed toward the energy channels ("meridians") and uses physical touch with pressure applied by a therapist and massage to address our pain experience. Acupressure works particularly well with muscle tension (e.g. spasms and trigger points) as it affects circulation and nerves, but certainly is not limited to exclusively treating muscles. Again the focus is on removing interference to the natural functioning of the body's energy system as an avenue to pain reduction.

---

10   Lymph is a clear fluid that transports waste materials through the body.

Stretching and Movement

There are physical forms of movement and stretching that are designed to move the flow of energy in the body, which can have cardiovascular, as well as muscular and nervous system benefits. Such movements can be valuable in increasing our range of motion, and strength using a gentle approach that allows us to be sensitive to our pain, while also challenging us to be as active as possible. We can extend our abilities while decreasing our overall pain intensity levels.

- *Hatha Yoga*...a discipline utilizing a series of specific physical postures of increasing levels of difficulty, which gently stretch the body's muscle, groups. It is often done in synchronization with the breath. In fact there are a series of very detailed breathing practices outlined in Yoga. Breath is considered a vital source of energy (called *prana*).
- *Tai Chi*..."Chi" is life force or energy. Tai Chi is many things, but for our purposes, it is an active form of meditation that resembles a slow motion ballet. It originated as a martial art, but was developed as an advanced form that uses the flow of energy in the body to quiet mind and spirit. If your range of motion is limited, this is an excellent, gentle movement form that allows you to go at your own pace and increase, or at least maintain your range of motion. In fact it accomplishes this so well that the Lupus Foundation of America, Inc. uses a video entitled the "ROM Dance", which is actually an adaptation of Tai Chi, as part of its educational training program for Lupus patients.
- *Qi Gong*...QiGong, pronounced "Chee Gung", is another form of slow and gentle movement. The focus remains on energy, but the goal is a bit different. QiGong

concentrates on *gathering* energy, whereas Tai Chi is more focused on circulating energy. Its origins come from the healing arts rather than the martial arts. This is not to say that the two are opposed to each other…in fact they nicely complement each other…but there are some differences. QiGong may be practiced sitting or standing, or lying down, as well as while moving. The gathered energy, it is affirmed, naturally seeks out obstruction to its flow, and removes these obstructions. It is used as preventative medicine as well as for healing. The varieties of problems it is used to address are vast.

Biofeedback

Biofeedback is a method of learning to self-regulate some of the body's physical systems, which normally tend to run on autopilot. We might, for example, monitor heart rate or circulation. Muscle tension in specific areas of the body is often monitored as well. We receive audio and visual feedback as measurements are taken on these various systems. The feedback tells us whether we're hitting the mark as we attempt to influence a specific system. Perhaps a tone signals that we're decreasing muscle tension in an area that tends to spasm uncomfortably. It is essentially a learning tool that facilitates our ability to use imagination and concentration to effect physical changes. The feedback validates our efforts. We don't have to wonder about whether we are *really* warming our hands (a good treatment for hypertension or headache)…we have the feedback. We are even beginning to learn how to alter brainwave patterns to provide relief for chronic conditions varying from depression to pain. Biofeedback is also widely used for stress management.

Miscellaneous

- *Pain management specialists* (often physicians that specialize in anesthesiology) use a variety of techniques to manage pain. These include *injections* to inhibit nerve impulses (nerve blocks), *physically implanting* electrical stimulation devices and implanting pumps that deliver certain medications directly to the spinal region, and *surgical* procedures for a great variety of medical problems.

- *Medication* is, of course, a treatment available for pain remediation. While most effective with acute pain, it can also be quite helpful with chronic discomfort as well. There is the possibility of your body becoming accustomed to some types of medication over time (called *tolerance*). Increasingly larger doses are then required to achieve equivalent results. This needs to be closely monitored, but needn't frighten you away. You simply need to consult with your physician on this matter.

- *Heat* can often be relaxing, and relieve muscle tension. The *dry* heat of an electrical heating pad is helpful for some. *Wet* heat is more helpful for others. Wet heat can be gotten by taking a hot bath or shower, and there are also a variety of heat packs that also provide moist heat (some are heated in a microwave oven and others are electrically maintained). One other method is a *paraffin* (that's right...wax) bath. This is used for hands and elbows for instance. Paraffin does a good job of insulating and enclosing the heat.

Conclusion

This listing can give you a sense of some of the options available to you. You should consult with your health care specialist...physician, nurse, physical therapist, etc. as you decide what's best for you. And let me again emphasize that the options I've presented here are only a cross section of the available pain management devices and techniques. This should help you initiate an informed exploration.

How We Change
Opposition and Conflict

There is a common thread that weaves through this book, and I wanted to leave you with a general view…even a worldview, which can inform your choices. The point of my emphasis on attitude has been based on my conviction that if we have "Got our minds right", then the details will follow. I trust our creative, healing instincts to guide us in the right direction, if the proper principles are applied.

My undergraduate training was in philosophy, not psychology. I found myself leaning toward two major traditions: Greek and Chinese. I also had a passion for theology both Eastern and Western. As I moved into the counseling field, I found a theme that coincided with my philosophy training. I have become a student of change and flexible adaptation. I constantly wonder about how we effect lasting changes in attitude and behavior. I conclude that *balance* is central to this project.

We have noted on numerous occasions (practically chapter by chapter) the problem that traveling in the land of the extreme creates. Too fast vs. too slow; Perfection vs. Failure; Worthy vs. Worthless; Overextended vs. Lazy; Happy vs. Sad; Acceptance vs. Denial; Avoidance vs. Confrontation are just some of the conflicts we've encountered. The dynamic of opposites mirroring each other on our journey of adjustment, recovery, and healing, is what informs us about the strategy that can lead to useful and productive change. As we learn how to live with our ongoing injury or illness and the attendant limitations and symptoms, we begin to find the balance between the extremes. As I mentioned above, the details will evolve from our attitudes.

Wait and See

We discover that it is possible to live in a world that *includes* the opposite extremes. We needn't ride a perpetual roller coaster of dramatic shifts…be they emotional, perceptual, or attitudinal. The inclusive "both/and" (as opposed to "either/or") outlook can, and will, level things out quite nicely. Each situation calls for its own creative, spontaneous response. This need not relegate us to a relativistic morality that erases the boundaries between right and wrong. No, in fact, it can liberate us.

This creative spontaneity allows for flexibility, for a gentle and accurate response to whatever circumstances we encounter. We will actually be able to most effectively and consistently apply our values.

We should avoid the tendency to become rigid. To say, "Don't get your hopes up" needn't mean, "Things probably won't work out". Rather it simply encourages us to approach events with a watchful and receptive expectancy. "Wait and see" is a more useful interpretation. This *descriptive* attitude does not make value judgments that often exclude much valuable information. Value judgments are excluded because after we assign a negative label (e.g. *bad*) to something, we will tend to either avoid it or discount it. It gets thrown out with the garbage because it's trash; it has no value and should be eliminated. Description, by contrast, is not hasty and does not go to the extreme. All information is potentially valuable. In fact we will often learn more from the socalled *negatives*, because they're usually the warning signs that, if identified, allow us to "nip it in the bud" and address problems before they become disasters.

Awareness

Where do we begin in the process of change and adjustment? Awareness is the first step. Initially we must be conscious of the pattern of thinking, behaving, or perceiving that requires change and revision. We need to develop the habit of "catching ourselves" in counterproductive, self-defeating patterns. To do so we must (a) be able to spot that pattern, and (b) acknowledge that the pattern isn't working. We can let the rule of balance in conjunction with our judgment regarding outcomes guide our assessment.

Chances are that if we're going to the extremes, the outcomes can bear to be improved upon. Thus watching for extreme patterns of thought and action is a good starting point in developing our ability to catch ourselves. Suspicion, for example, may make trust impossible…or a daylong project done without breaks may put us in bed the following day. Let's assume that we have negotiated this piece of work. What next?

Staging the Process

If we're perceiving, thinking, or doing things differently half the time, we've made an excellent start! I would therefore recommend that we set a difference of 50% as our initial goal for effecting change. Our progress will continue, if we remain focused and attentive. It may not happen as quickly as we would like; we may not be able to predict *when* change will occur, but we will find that persistence virtually guarantees success.

We need to make sure we're doing *our* part. We can catch our cynicism, and be prepared to trust, but we cannot *make* ourselves trust. We can educate our family, but we cannot *make* them understand. The day will be much more relaxed if we just pay attention to what we're doing, to our responsibilities, which is what we actually *can* control. Of course, we need to see results, but we also need to be patient and deliberate. When we are deciding whether the change is a success and worth the effort, we need to give it time to adequately develop.

If we are able to maintain this focus, then we can feel good about achieving a 50 percent difference even though, for the present, it may not be "different enough" to suit us. We can also look forward to more improvement over time. Remember: "Progress, not perfection" is our dictum. We're taking incremental, graduated steps. Others may not credit our effort or success until we've been doing it for several months. There may be no acknowledgement until we're behaving differently *most* of the time (i.e., approaching 85 percent of the time). If the change is one of new perspective and perception, the rewards of serenity or insight may not show up for what may seem like an eternity. But keep in mind that this is definitely possible. I see this happen again and again with my clients. Persist! It *will* be worth it! And remember our sights are set on more good days than bad days. Even with a majority of good days, there will still be some bad days too.

The Garden

We used the image of the garden in the first chapter as an analogy to illustrate the concept of readiness. Well, we've come full circle as we conclude using the garden analogy to clarify our understanding of personal change. Change occurs in our life much like the flower blooms in the garden. We cultivate the soil by watering, weeding, and fertilizing. After all that care and attention, one morning, awaiting us when we awake, is the flower's bloom! We cannot accurately predict that morning, although we may be able to see some early indications of that day. Change is much the same for us. We can cultivate the garden, but cannot *make* the flower bloom…neither can we *make* ourselves accept our limitations. The change may appear as a dramatic overnight transformation, but time effort, and readiness are all important factors leading to that moment. Balance, once again, is and important factor. Over-watering is just as deadly as under-watering. Too much fertilizer is just as harmful as too little. Similarly it is possible to try too hard to change a habit of thinking or behaving. If we, for example, typically exercise very little, we will probably find that after a few weeks or months of daily, extended workouts, we quit altogether and revert to our sedentary lifestyle. Twenty minutes of daily exercise, or an hour every other day might have worked better…our chances of persisting might have been markedly better.

We don't want to uproot the potential flower while we're weeding the garden. Consider stubborn pride as an example. Pride can be useful, if harnessed and directed toward choosing to go beyond *surviving* the challenges of our illness, injury, or pain to, in fact, *thriving* as we utilize challenge to grow and mature.

It's just the right combination of all these ingredients that yields the healthy plant. And let us not forget to take the weather into account.

There are always those unknown variables to be factored into each day we work toward our goals, each day we cope with our illness/injury. It may be the behavior of another, or a twist of circumstance, that will demand our creative response.

Successful adjustments in our healing journey require balanced expectations, both of the process of change and of the long-term outcomes. There are limits to what can be accomplished, as there are limits to our ability to control and influence how and when the results will show up. But as we are able to persist, we *will* experience the rewards. Joy and satisfaction can be ours!

Summary

- Developing new skills enhances our ability to enjoy life.
- The proper outlook will give rise to useful coping strategies.
- The perspective that can integrate opposite extremes is the key to creative freedom and flexibility.
- A descriptive wait and see attitude gives us the largest information base from which to work.
- Understanding the nature of human change can help us choose moderation and maintain persistent effort.
- Awareness of self-defeating patterns of thought and action is where change begins.
- Lasting change is typically incremental…one step at a time.
- Effecting change is much like cultivating a garden.
- The bloom of change may appear overnight, but we must not forget the time and effort required prior to that final transformation.
- Change may seem miraculous, and in some way is an act of grace, but we bear the responsibility for balanced effort and persistence.

This book is INTERACTIVE…

To get access to additional resources to complement what is offered in this chapter visit…

http://michaelgusac.odgi.net/MYBK12

A FINAL WORD

THE JOURNEY NEVER really ends. As you complete this book, it is my hope that you have found at least three or four items that can be useful to you in your recovery. Healing and recovery is a dynamic process. And assuming that this is true, then our adjustment to our illness or injury is a life-long project. Think of this as a beginning. No matter how good we get at this, there will be good days and bad. This applies to our coping abilities as well as to our symptoms, to our energy level, as well as to our attitude.

My wife asked me early on in the writing of this book if it "felt good" to finally write it. I've been talking about writing it ever since my recovery began from Guillain-Barré Syndrome seven years ago. It occurs to me that this project has helped me better organize and understand my own recovery, even as it has given me the opportunity to share my perspective. I mention this to highlight the fact that we never really stop dealing with our illness or injury. The symptoms may wax and wane, but for many of us the symptomatic reminders, and the possibility of relapse and progressive deterioration of our condition keep us company through the years.

This book was written to get you started on the road to reclaiming your Self, your health…your life. It can also be a reference point to which you can return for a friendly reminder from time to time. Preventive maintenance requires ongoing awareness. That is why I want to encourage you to commit yourself to growth and learning in your adjustment to your illness or injury. The natural order of life is growth and development. To become rigid and inflexible is what will make you old before your time. When we're dealing with a chronic condition, life is already sufficiently challenging. Don't complicate it further. Don't become overly confident and decide you've got your recovery completely figured out. The Greek philosopher Socrates rightly declared that *wisdom* begins with our awareness of our *ignorance*, of how little we really know. Humility can refine our understanding and help us maintain a reasonable level of attentiveness. We needn't be looking over our shoulders all the time. But neither do we want to be making a habit of putting on our blinders.

You may well have come to the conclusion that many of the attitudes set forth in this book would be fairly useful in general, regardless of whether you have a chronic illness or injury. If so, that would certainly reinforce the value of these attitudes. You may have guessed that happens to be my view. When we are able to understand the limits of our control, we also begin to understand the range of our responsibilities. When the focus of our vision expands, we begin to realize that self-pity and worry are a fruitless waste. This has always been true, but our injury or illness crystallizes this awareness.

You may find yourself thinking "Nobody in their right mind would wish for this, but I have learned a lot." If left to our own devices, we would never have come to these insights, or have made the changes in attitude that we have made. Circumstances have forced us to confront our Self, and our beliefs. If we have learned well, our illness/injury will mature us in ways that will be fully understood only by those of us that have "been there", and then only as we look back on the challenges over an extended period of time. We may conclude that, in the larger view, there was a "reason" for the challenge, and that we are not only grateful for what we still have, but that we have also come to appreciate the journey. I know that's a bit of a stretch, but you may surprise yourself. There is hope! There is joy! And we don't have to wait for it. We can reach out and grasp it now!

As I work at the clinic or in my practice, I characteristically ask my clients what has most helped them in their recovery. Here are a few samples:

> "[I've learned that] my pain and I have to work together. I listen to it, and it listens to me. We're on the same team finally. Whereas before I tried to drag the 'sucker' into the mud hole; I was fighting with it; now I'm not." (Injured Fireman…age:mid-50's)

> "I had to change my attitude from negative to positive. I've learned to handle the pain some. I get up and I move. I try to focus on something else. Sometimes I call my daughter, and ask her to bring over my grandson." (Injured Cook…age:early-60's)

> "[What helped was] knowing that I had to accept it; [knowing] that I had to do something for myself." (Injured Construction Contractor…age: late-40's)

It is overly simplistic to suggest that there is merely one attitude that can adequately facilitate our healing, our recovery. But we will be able to identify that certain choices were the "turning point" for us. And notice here that I said decision. As we review the above statements, notice the underlying assumption…that these adjustments, these healing strategies, are decisions for change. We choose, at some point to change gears, stop fighting, become more positive, accept and nurture ourselves as these men and women have done. Difficult choices, but well worth it. The rewards are immeasurable, and often beyond what we can put into words. The effects encompass our entire being at the deepest levels…not only intellect, but also body and soul. And the journey does not end here…It begins!

Be well.

If you've enjoyed this book, please leave a review of it on Amazon, which can be done by following this link:

https://www.amazon.com/dp/B076Z34J9W

Thank you so much!

ABOUT THE AUTHOR

MICHAEL GUSACK, MA was diagnosed with a chronic kidney condition over 17 years ago. Ten years ago he was diagnosed with Guillain Barre' Syndrome which is a condition that affects the central and peripheral nervous system.

He is nationally certified in Biofeedback and Hypnosis, Sports Counseling, Addictions, and Medical Qigong. A psychotherapist for over 25 years, his involvement with meditation, yoga, Tai Chi, and Qigong has prepared him well to blend the complementary Eastern and Western healing traditions in a way that has empowered thousands to regain control of their lives as they develop the skills and attitudes that best facilitate life's opportunities for joy and satisfaction.

His hospitalization with Guillain Barre' Syndrome planted the seed that has developed into this book. The message here goes far beyond the confines of medical illness per se', since it applies to pain that is spiritual, as well as physical in nature.

His current practice and interests allow him to push the clinical envelope. He works with biofeedback to facilitate and refine relaxation, meditation, and healing visualizations relative to managing physical and spiritual pain. He is exploring the potential benefits of brain-wave feedback. New treatment modalities such as work with photo-sonic stimulation, low frequency sound wave massage (based on research gleaned from studies of Chinese Qigong healing masters), and microcurrent stimulation are also part of his daily practice. He was recently certified in Medical Qigong.

Michael was born in Wiesbaden, Germany. He now lives with his wife of over 25 years and his 12 and 16-year-old daughters in Gulf Breeze, Florida where he bases his private practice. He specializes in pain and illness management, stress management, and performance enhancement training.

RESOURCES

Alberti, Robert E., and Emmons, Michael. *Your Perfect Right*. San Luis Obispo, California: Impact Press, 1974.

Aristotle. The Metaphysics. 28th ed. Translated by W.D. Ross in The Basic Works of Aristotle. Edited by Richard McKeon. New York: Random House,1941.

Barasch, Marc Ian. The Healing Path: A Soul Approach to Illness. New York: Tarcher/ Putnam Book by G.P. Putnam's Sons, 1993.

Benson, Herbert. *The Relaxation Response*. New York: William Morrow, 1975

Borysenko, Joan. *Minding the Body, Mending the Mind*. Reading ,MA: Addison-Wesley, 1987.

Casarjian, Robin. *Forgiveness: A Bold Choice for a Peaceful Heart.*. New York: Bantam Books, 1992.

Caudill, Margaret. *Managing Pain Before It Manages You*. New York: The Guilford Press, 1995.

Cousins, Norman. *Anatomy of an Illness*. New York: Bantam Books, 1981. Davis, Martha; Eschelman, Elizabeth and McKay, Matthew. *The Relaxation and Stress Reduction Workbook*. Oakland, CA: New Harbinger, 1988.

Descartes, Rene'. *Meditations on First Philosophy*. Translated by Norman

Kemp Smith in *Descartes: Philosophical Writings*, New York: Modern Library, 1958.

Dossey, Larry. *Healing Words: The Power Of Prayer And The Practice Of Medicine*. San Francisco: Harper Collins, 1993.

Ellis, Albert, and Greiger, Russell. *Handbook of Rational Emotive Therapy*. New York: Springer, 1977.

Gold, Mark S. *The Good News About Panic, Anxiety, and Phobias*. New York: Bantam Books, 1990.

Goode, Ruth, and Sussman, Aaron. *The Magic of Walking*. New York: Simon and Shuster, 1967.

Gray, Henry. *Anatomy, Descriptive and Surgical*. Edited by T. Pickering Pick, and Robert Howden. New York: Gramercy Books, 1977.

Herbert, Frank. Dune. New York: The Putnam Publishing Group, 1984. Jacobson, Edmund. *Progressive Relaxation*. Chicago: University of Chicago Press, 1938.

Kabat-Zinn, John. *Full Catastrophe Living: Using the Wisdom of Your Body and Mind to Face Stress, Pain and Illness*. New York: Delacorte Press, 1990.

Luthe, Wolfgang. "Autogenic Training: Method, Research and Application in Medicine." *American Journal of Psychotherapy*. 1963, vol. 17, 174-95. Melzack, Ronald, and Wall, Patrick D. *The Challenge of Pain: Exciting Discoveries in the New Science of Pain Control*. New York: Basic Books,1983.

Ornstein, Robert. *The Psychology of Consciousness*. San Francisco: W. H. Freeman & Company, 1972.

Pelletier, Kenneth R. *Mind as healer, Mind as Slayer*. New York: Delta, 1977. Plato. *The Symposium*. Translated by Walter Hamilton. Baltimore,

Maryland: Penguin Books, Inc., 1971.

Selye, Hans. *Stress Without Distress*. New York: Dutton, 1974.

Shealy, C. Norman. *90 Days to Self-Health*. New York: Dial Press, 1977. Siegel, Bernie S. *Love, Medicine, and Miracles*. New York: Harper & Row, 1977.

Simon, Sidney B., and Simon, Suzanne. *Forgiveness: How To Make Peace With Your Past And Get On With Your Life.* New York: Warner Books, 1990.

Suzuki, Shunryu. *Zen Mind, Beginner's Mind.* New York: Weatherhill, 1970.

Tse, Michael. *Qigong For Health & Vitality.* New York: St. Martin's Press, 1996.

Weil, Andrew. *Spontaneous Healing: How to Discover and Enhance Your Body's Natural Ability to Maintain and Heal Itself.* New York: Knopf Publishing Group,1995.

Wilhelm, Helmut. *Change.* Translated by Cary F. Baynes. Princeton, New Jersey: Princeton University Press, 1960.

www.ingramcontent.com/pod-product-compliance
Lightning Source LLC
Chambersburg PA
CBHW070237230526
45470CB00002B/447